Statistics Explained

Statistics Explained is a reader-friendly introduction to experimental design and statistics for undergraduate students in the life sciences, particularly those who do not have a strong mathematical background. Hypothesis testing and experimental design are discussed first. Statistical tests are then explained using pictorial examples and a minimum of formulae. This class-tested approach, along with a well-structured set of diagnostic tables, will give students the confidence to choose an appropriate test with which to analyse their own data sets. Presented in a lively and straightforward manner *Statistics Explained* will give readers the depth and background necessary to proceed to more advanced texts and applications. It will therefore be essential reading for all bioscience undergraduates, and will serve as a useful refresher course for more advanced students.

Steve McKillup is an Associate Professor of Biology in the School of Biological and Environmental Sciences at Central Queensland University, Rockhampton.

Statistics Explained

An Introductory Guide for Life Scientists

STEVE McKILLUP

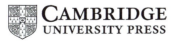
CAMBRIDGE
UNIVERSITY PRESS

9-29-2006
WW
$29.99

CAMBRIDGE UNIVERSITY PRESS
Cambridge, New York, Melbourne, Madrid, Cape Town, Singapore, São Paulo

CAMBRIDGE UNIVERSITY PRESS
The Edinburgh Building, Cambridge CB2 2RU, UK

www.cambridge.org
Information on this title: www.cambridge.org/9780521835503

First published 2006

Printed in the United Kingdom at the University Press, Cambridge

A catalogue record for this publication is available from the British Library

ISBN-13 978-0-521-83550-3 hardback
ISBN-10 0-521-83550-X hardback

ISBN-13 978-0-521-54316-3 paperback
ISBN-10 0-521-54316-9 paperback

Contents

Preface

If you mention 'statistics' or 'biostatistics' to life scientists, they often look nervous. Many fear or dislike mathematics, but an understanding of statistics and experimental design is essential for graduates, postgraduates, and researchers in the biological, biochemical, health, and human movement sciences.

Since this understanding is so important, life science students are usually made to take some compulsory undergraduate statistics courses. Nevertheless, I found that a lot of graduates (and postgraduates) were unsure about designing experiments and had difficulty knowing which statistical test to use (and which ones not to!) when analysing their results. Some even told me they had found statistics courses 'boring, irrelevant and hard to understand'.

It seemed there was a problem with the way many introductory biostatistics courses were presented, which was making students disinterested and preventing them from understanding the concepts needed to progress to higher-level courses and more complex statistical applications. There seemed to be two major reasons for this problem, and as a student I encountered both.

First, a lot of statistics textbooks take a mathematical approach and often launch into considerable detail and pages of daunting looking formulae without any straightforward explanation about what statistical testing really does.

Second, introductory biostatistics courses are often taught in a way that does not cater for life science students who may lack a strong mathematical background.

When I started teaching at Central Queensland University I thought there had to be a better way of introducing essential concepts of biostatistics and experimental design. It had to start from first principles and develop an understanding that could be applied to all statistical tests. It had to demystify what these tests actually did and explain them with a minimum of formulae and terminology. It had to relate statistical concepts to experimental design. And, finally, it had to build a strong understanding to help the student progress to more complex material. I tried this approach with my undergraduate classes and the response from a lot of students, including some postgraduates who sat in on the course, was, 'Hey Steve, you should write an introductory stats book!'

Ward Cooper suggested I submit a proposal for this sort of book to Cambridge University Press. Ruth McKillup read, commented on, and reread several drafts, provided constant encouragement, and tolerated my absent mindedness. My students, especially Steve Dunbar, Kevin Strychar, and Glenn Druery, encouraged me to start writing and my friends and colleagues, especially Dearne Mayer and Sandy Dalton, encouraged me to finish. Finally, I sincerely thank the anonymous reviewers of the initial proposal and the subsequent manuscript who, without exception, made most appropriate suggestions for improvement.

1 | Introduction

1.1 Why do life scientists need to know about experimental design and statistics?

If you work on living things it is usually impossible to get data from every individual of the group or species in question. Imagine trying to measure the length of every anchovy in the Pacific Ocean, the haemoglobin count of every adult in the USA, the diameter of every pine tree in a plantation of 200 000, or the individual protein content of 10 000 prawns in a large aquaculture pond.

The total number of individuals of a particular species present in a defined area is often called the **population**. Since a researcher usually cannot measure every individual in the population (unless they are studying the few remaining members of an endangered species), they have to work with a carefully selected **subset** containing several individuals, often called **experimental units,** that they hope is a **representative sample** from which the characteristics of the population can be inferred. You can also think of a population as the total number of artificial experimental units possible (e.g. the 125 567 plots of 1 m^2 that would cover a coral reef) and your sample being the subset (e.g. 20 plots) you have chosen to work with.

The best way to get a representative sample is usually to choose a proportion of the population at **random** – without bias, with every possible experimental unit having an equal chance of being selected.

The trouble with this approach is that there are often great differences among experimental units from the same population. Think of the people you have seen today – unless you met some identical twins (or triplets etc.), no two would have been the same. Even species that seem to be made up of similar looking individuals (like flies or cockroaches or snails) show great variability. This leads to several problems.

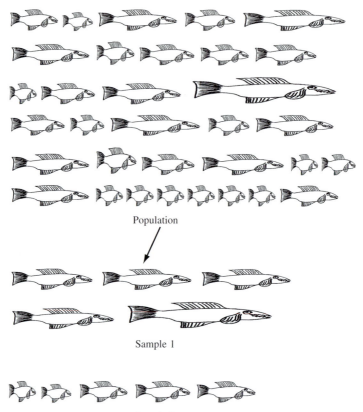

Population

Sample 1

Sample 2

Figure 1.1   Even a random sample may not necessarily be a good representative of the population. Two samples have been taken at random from the same population. By chance, sample 1 contains a group of relatively large fish, while those in sample 2 are relatively small.

First, even a random sample may not be a good representative of the population from which it has been taken (Figure 1.1). For example, you may choose students for an exercise experiment who are, by chance, far less (or far more) physically fit than the population of the college they represent; a batch of seed chosen at random may not represent the variability present in all seed of that species; and a sample of mosquitoes from a particular place may have very different insecticide resistance than the same species from elsewhere.

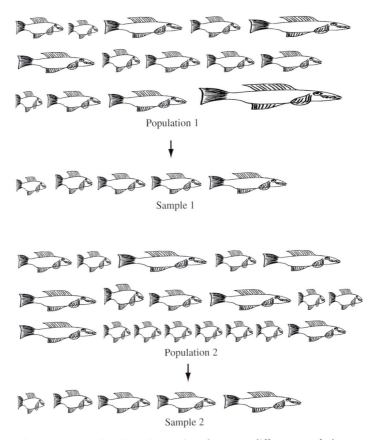

Figure 1.2 Samples selected at random from very different populations may not necessarily be different. Simply by chance sample 1 and sample 2 are similar.

Therefore, **if you take a random sample from each of two similar populations, the samples may be different to each other simply by chance.** On the basis of this you might mistakenly conclude that the two populations are very different. You need some way of knowing if the difference between samples is one you would expect by chance, or whether the populations really do seem to be different.

Second, even if two populations are very different, samples from each may be similar, and give the misleading impression the populations are also similar (Figure 1.2).

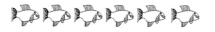

Control group (before the experiment)

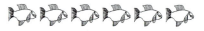

Treatment group (before the experiment)

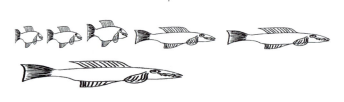

Control group (after 300 days)

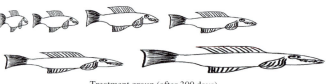

Treatment group (after 300 days)

Figure 1.3 Two samples of fish were taken from the same population and deliberately matched so that six equal-sized individuals were initially present in each group. Fish in the treatment group were fed a vitamin supplement for 300 days, while those in the untreated control group were not. The supplement caused each fish in the treatment group to grow about 10% longer, but this difference is small compared with the variation in growth among individuals, which may obscure any effect of treatment.

Finally, natural variation among individuals within a sample may obscure any effect of an experimental treatment (Figure 1.3). There is often so much variation within a sample (and a population) that an effect of treatment may be difficult or impossible to detect. For example, what would you conclude if you found that 50 people given a newly synthesised drug showed an average decrease in blood pressure, but when you looked more closely at the group you found that blood pressure remained unchanged for 25, decreased markedly for 15, and increased slightly for the remaining 10? Has the drug really had an effect? What if tomato plants treated with a new fertiliser yielded from 1.5 to 9 kg of fruit per plant, compared with 1.5 to 7.5 kg per plant in an untreated group? Would you conclude there was a meaningful difference between these two groups?

These sorts of problems are usually unavoidable when you work with samples and mean that a researcher has to take every possible precaution to try and ensure their samples are likely to be **representative** and thus give a good estimate of conditions in the population. Researchers need to know how to sample. They also need a good understanding of experimental design, because a good design will take natural variation into account and also minimise additional unwanted variation introduced by the experimental procedure itself. They also need to take accurate and precise measurements to minimise other sources of error.

Finally, considering the variability among samples described above, the results of an experiment may not be clear-cut. So it is often difficult to make a decision about a difference between samples from different populations or different experimental treatments. **Is it the sort of difference you would expect by chance, or are the populations really different? Is the experimental treatment having an effect?**

You need something to **help you decide**, and that is what statistical tests do, by calculating the probability of obtaining a particular difference among samples. Once you have the probability, the decision is up to you. So you need to understand how statistical tests work!

1.2 What is this book designed to do?

An understanding of experimental design and statistics is important, whether you are a biomedical scientist, ecologist, entomologist, genetic engineer, microbiologist, nursing professional, taxonomist, or human movement scientist, so most life science students are made to take a general introductory statistics course. Many of these courses take a detailed mathematical approach that a lot of life scientists find uninspiring. This book is an introduction that does not assume a strong mathematical background. Instead, it develops a conceptual understanding of how statistical tests actually work, using pictorial explanations where possible and a minimum of formulae.

If you have read other texts, or have already done an introductory course, you may find that the way this material is presented is unusual, but I have found that non-statisticians find this approach very easy to understand and sometimes even entertaining. If you have a background in statistics you may find some sections a little too explanatory, but at the same time they are likely to make sense. This book most certainly will not teach you everything about the subject areas, but it will help you decide what sort of statistical test to use and what the results mean. It will also help you understand and criticise the experimental designs of others. Most importantly, it will help you design and analyse your own experiments, understand more complex experimental designs, and move on to more advanced statistical courses.

2 | 'Doing science' – hypotheses, experiments, and disproof

2.1   Introduction

Before starting on experimental design and statistics, it is important to be familiar with how science is done. This is a summary of a very conventional view of scientific method.

2.2   Basic scientific method

The essential features of the 'hypothetico-deductive' view of scientific method (see Popper, 1968) are that a person observes or samples the natural world and uses all the information available to make an intuitive, logical guess, called an **hypothesis**, about how the system functions. The person has no way of knowing if their hypothesis is correct – it may or may not apply. **Predictions** made from the hypothesis are tested, either by further sampling or by doing experiments. If the results are consistent with the predictions then the hypothesis is retained. If they are not, it is rejected, and a new hypothesis formulated (Figure 2.1).

The initial hypothesis may come about as a result of observations, sampling, and/or reading the scientific literature. Here is an example from ecological entomology.

The Portuguese millipede *Ommatioulus moreleti* was accidentally introduced into southern Australia from Portugal in the 1950s. This millipede lives in leaf litter and grows to about four centimetres long. In the absence of natural enemies from its country of origin (especially European hedgehogs, which eat a lot of millipedes), its numbers rapidly increased to plague proportions in South Australia. Although it causes very little damage to agricultural crops, *O. moreleti* is a serious 'nuisance' pest because it invades houses. In heavily infested areas of South Australia during the late 1980s it

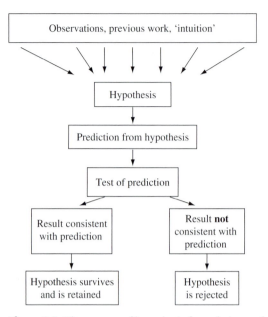

Figure 2.1 The process of hypothesis formulation and testing.

used to be common to find over 1000 millipedes invading a moderate sized house in just one night. When you disturb one of these millipedes it ejects a smelly yellow defensive secretion. Once inside a house the millipedes would crawl across the floor, up the walls, and over the ceiling, where they fell into food and on to the faces and even into the open mouths of sleeping people. When accidentally crushed underfoot they stained carpets and floors, and smelt. The problem was so great that almost half a million dollars was spent on research to control this pest.

While working on ways to reduce the nuisance caused by the Portuguese millipede I noticed that householders who reported severe problems had well-lit houses with large, uncurtained windows. In contrast, nearby neighbours whose houses were not so well lit, and who closed their curtains at night, reported far fewer millipedes inside. The numbers of *O. moreleti* per square metre were similar in the leaf litter around both types of houses. From these observations and very limited sampling of less than ten houses, I formulated the hypothesis, 'Portuguese millipedes are attracted to visible light at night.' I had no way of knowing whether this simple hypothesis was the reason for home invasions by millipedes, but it seemed logical from my observations.

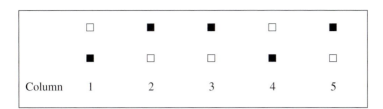

Figure 2.2 Arrangement of a 2 × 5 grid of lit and unlit tiles across a field where millipedes were abundant. Filled squares indicate unlit tiles and open squares indicate lit tiles.

From this hypothesis it was straightforward to predict, 'At night, in a field where Portuguese millipedes are abundant, more will be present on white tiles illuminated by visible light than on unlit white tiles.'

This prediction was tested by doing a simple and inexpensive manipulative field experiment with two treatments – lit tiles and a control treatment of unlit tiles.

Since any difference in millipede numbers between one lit and one unlit tile might occur just by chance or some other unknown factor(s), the two treatments were **replicated** five times. I set up ten identical white ceramic floor tiles in a two row × five column rectangular grid in a field where millipedes were abundant (Figure 2.2). For each column of two tiles, I tossed a coin to decide which of the pair was going to be lit. The other tile was left unlit. Having one lit tile in each column ensured that replicates of both the treatment and control were dispersed across the field rather than having all the treatment tiles clustered together and was a precaution in case the number of millipedes per square metre varied across the field. The coin tossing eliminated any likelihood that I might subconsciously place the lit tile of each pair in an area where millipedes were more common.

I hammered a thin two metre long wooden stake vertically into the ground next to each tile. For every one of the lit tiles I attached a pocket torch to its stake and made sure the light shone on the tile.

I started the experiment at dusk by turning on the torches. Three hours later I went back and counted the numbers of millipedes on all tiles. The tiles within each treatment were the experimental units (Chapter 1).

From this experiment there were at least four possible outcomes:

1 No millipedes were present on the unlit tiles but lots were present on each of the lit tiles. This result is consistent with the hypothesis, which has survived this initial test and can be retained.

2 High and similar numbers of millipedes were present on both the lit and unlit tiles. This is not consistent with the hypothesis, which can probably be rejected since it seems light has no effect.

3 No (or very few) millipedes were present on any tiles. It is difficult to know if this has any bearing on the hypothesis – there may be a fault with the experiment (e.g. the tiles were themselves repellent or perhaps too slippery, or millipedes may not have been active that night). The hypothesis is neither rejected nor retained.

4 Lots of millipedes were present on the unlit tiles, but none were present on the lit ones. This is a most unexpected outcome that is not consistent with the hypothesis, which is extremely likely to be rejected.

These are the four simplest outcomes. A more complicated and much more likely one is that you find **some** millipedes on the tiles in **both** treatments, and that is what happened – see McKillup (1988). This sort of outcome is a problem, because you need to decide if light is having an effect on the millipedes, or whether the difference in numbers between lit and unlit treatments is simply **happening by chance**. Here statistical testing is extremely useful and necessary because it helps you decide whether a difference between treatments is meaningful.

2.3   Making a decision about an hypothesis

Once you have the result of the experimental test of an hypothesis, two things can happen:

either the results of the experiment are consistent with the hypothesis, which is retained;

or the results are inconsistent with the hypothesis, which may be rejected.

If the hypothesis is rejected it is likely to be wrong and another will need to be proposed.

If the hypothesis is retained, withstands further testing, and has some very widespread generality, it may progress to become a **theory**. But a theory is only ever a very general hypothesis that has withstood repeated testing. There is always a possibility it may be disproven in the future.

2.4   Why can't an hypothesis or theory ever be proven?

No hypothesis or theory can ever be proven – one day there may be evidence that rejects it and leads to a different explanation (which can include all the successful predictions of the previous hypothesis). Consequently we can only falsify or disprove hypotheses and theories – we can never ever prove them.

Cases of disproof and a subsequent change in thinking are common. Here are two examples.

Medical researchers used to believe that excess stomach acidity was responsible for the majority of gastric ulcers in humans. There was a radical change in thinking when many ulcers healed following antibiotic therapy designed to reduce numbers of the bacterium *Helicobacter pylori* in the stomach wall.

There have been at least three theories of how the human kidney produces a concentrated solution of urine, and the latest may not necessarily be correct.

2.5   'Negative' outcomes

People are often quite disappointed if the outcome of an experiment is not what they expected and their hypothesis is rejected. But there is nothing wrong with this – rejection of an hypothesis is still progress in the process of understanding how a system functions. Therefore, a 'negative' outcome that causes you to reject a cherished hypothesis is just as important as a 'positive' one that causes you to retain it.

Unfortunately researchers tend to be very possessive and protective of their hypotheses, and there have been cases where results have been falsified in order to allow an hypothesis to survive. This does not advance our understanding of the world and is likely to be detected when other scientists repeat the experiments or do further experiments based on these false conclusions. There will be more about this in Chapter 20, which is about doing science responsibly and ethically.

2.6   Null and alternate hypotheses

It is scientific convention that when you test an hypothesis you state it as two hypotheses, which are essentially alternates. For example, the hypothesis, 'Portuguese millipedes are attracted to visible light at night', is usually stated in combination with, 'Portuguese millipedes are **not** attracted to visible light at night'. The latter includes all cases not included in the first hypothesis (e.g. no response, or avoidance of visible light).

These hypotheses are called the **alternate** and **null** hypotheses respectively. Importantly, the null hypothesis is always stated as the hypothesis of 'no difference' or 'no effect'. So, looking at the two hypotheses above, the second 'are not' hypothesis is the null hypothesis and the first is the alternate hypothesis. This is a tedious but very important convention (because it clearly states the hypothesis and its alternative) and there will be several reminders in this book.

Box 2.1 Two other views about scientific method

Popper's hypothetico-deductive philosophy of scientific method, where hypotheses are sequentially tested and always at risk of being rejected, is widely accepted. In reality, however, scientists may do things a little differently.

Kuhn (1970) argues that scientific enquiry does not necessarily proceed with the steady testing and survival or rejection of hypotheses. Instead, hypotheses with some generality and which have survived initial testing become well-established theories or 'paradigms', which are relatively immune to rejection even if subsequent testing may find evidence against them. A few negative results are used to refine the paradigm to make it continue to fit all available evidence. It is only when the negative evidence becomes overwhelming that the paradigm is rejected and replaced by a new one.

Lakatos (1978) also argues that a strict hypothetico-deductive process of scientific enquiry does not necessarily occur. Instead, fields of enquiry, called 'research programmes' are based on a set of 'core' theories that are rarely questioned or tested. The core is surrounded by a protective 'belt' of theories that are tested. A successful research programme is one that accumulates more and more theories that have survived testing within the belt, which provides increasing protection for the core. If, however, many of the belt theories are rejected, doubt will eventually be cast on the veracity of the core and of the research programme itself, which will be replaced by a more successful one.

These two views and the hypothetico-deductive view are not irreconcilable. In all cases observations and experiments provide evidence either for or against an hypothesis or theory. In the hypothetico-deductive view science proceeds by the orderly testing and survival or rejection of individual hypotheses, while the other two views reflect the complexity of theories required to describe a research area and emphasise that it would be foolish to reject a theory outright on the basis of limited negative evidence.

2.7   Conclusion

There are five components to an experiment: (1) formulating an hypothesis, (2) making a prediction from the hypothesis, (3) doing an experiment or sampling to test the prediction, (4) analysing the data, and (5) deciding whether to retain or reject the hypothesis.

The description of scientific method given here is extremely simple and basic and there has been an enormous amount of philosophical debate about how science is done (see Box 2.1). For example, more than one hypothesis might explain a set of observations and it may be difficult to test these by progressively considering each one against its null. For further reading, Chalmers (1999) gives a very readable and clearly explained discussion of the process and philosophy of scientific discovery.

3 | Collecting and displaying data

3.1 Introduction

One way of generating hypotheses is to collect data and look for patterns. Often, however, it is difficult to see any pattern from a set of data, which may just be a list of numbers. Graphs and descriptive statistics are very useful for summarising and displaying data in ways that may reveal patterns. This chapter describes the different types of data you are likely to encounter and discusses ways of displaying them.

3.2 Variables, experimental units, and types of data

The particular attributes you measure when you collect data are called **variables** (e.g. body temperature, the numbers of a particular species of beetle per broad bean pod, the amount of fungal damage per leaf, or the numbers of brown and albino mice). These data are collected from each experimental unit, which may be an individual (e.g. a human being or a whale) or a defined item (e.g. a square metre of the seabed, a leaf, or a lake). If you only measure one variable per experimental unit, the data set is **univariate**. Data for two variables per unit are **bivariate**, while data for three or more variables measured on the same experimental unit are **multivariate**.

Variables can be measured on four scales – ratio, interval, ordinal, or nominal.

A **ratio scale** describes a variable whose numerical values truly indicate the quantity being measured.

- There is a true zero point below which you cannot have any data (for example, if you are measuring the lengths of lizards, you cannot have a lizard of negative length).

- An increase of the same numerical amount indicates the same quantity across the range of measurements (for example, a 2 cm and a 40 cm lizard will have grown by the same amount, if they both increase in length by 10 cm).
- A particular ratio holds across the range of the variable (for example, a 40 cm lizard is 20 times longer than a 2 cm lizard and a 100 cm lizard is also 20 times longer than a 5 cm lizard).

An **interval scale** describes a variable that can be less than zero.

- The zero point is arbitrary (for example, temperature measured in degrees celsius has a zero point at which water freezes), so negative values are possible. The true zero point for temperature, where there is a complete absence of heat, is zero kelvin (about $-273°C$), so unlike the celsius scale the kelvin scale is a ratio scale.
- An increase of the same numerical amount indicates the same quantity across the range of measurements (for example a $2°C$ increase indicates the same increase in heat whatever the starting temperature).
- Since the zero point is arbitrary, a particular ratio does not hold across the range of the variable (for example, the ratio of $6°C$ compared with $1°C$ is not the same as $60°C$ with $10°C$. The two ratios in terms of the kelvin scale are 279 : 274 K and 333 : 283 K).

An **ordinal scale** applies to data where values are ranked – given a value that simply indicates their **relative order**. These ranks do not necessarily indicate constant differences. For example, five children of ages 2, 7, 9, 10, and 16 years have been aged on a ratio scale. If, however, you rank these ages in order from the youngest to the oldest (e.g. as ranks 1 to 5), the data have been reduced to an ordinal scale. Child 2 is not necessarily twice as old as child 1.

- An increase in the same numerical amount of ranks does not necessarily hold across the range of the variable.

A **nominal scale** applies to data where the values are classified according to an attribute. For example, if there are only two possible forms of coat colour in mice, then a sample of mice can be subdivided into the numbers within each of these two attributes.

The first three categories described above can include either **continuous** or **discrete** data. Nominal scale data (since they are attributes) can only be discrete.

Continuous data can have any value within a range. For example, any value of temperature is possible within the range from 10°C to 20°C, such as 15.3°C or 17.82°C.

Discrete data are very different to continuous data, because they can only have fixed numerical values within a range. For example, the number of offspring produced increases from one fixed whole number to the next, because you cannot have a fraction of an offspring.

It is important that you know what type of data you are dealing with, because this will be one of the factors that determines your choice of statistical test.

3.3   Displaying data

A list of data may reveal very little, but a pictorial summary is a way of exploring the data that might help you notice a pattern, which can help generate or test hypotheses.

3.3.1   Histograms

Here is a list of the number of visits made to a medical doctor during the previous six months by a sample of 60 students chosen at random from a first-year university biostatistics class of 600. These data are univariate, ratio scaled, and discrete:

1,11,2,1,10,2,1,1,1,1,12,1,6,2,1,2,2,7,1,2,1,1,1,1,1,3,1,2,1,2,1,4,6,9,1,2,8,1,9,1, 8,1,1,1,2, 2,1,2,1,2,1,1,8,1,2,1,1,1,1,7

It is difficult to see any pattern from this list of numbers, but you could summarise and display these data by drawing a histogram. To do this you separately count the number (the **frequency**) of cases for students who visited a medical doctor never, once, twice, three times, through to the maximum number of visits and plot these as a series of rectangles on a graph with the X axis showing the number of visits and the Y axis the number of students in each of these cases. Figure 3.1 shows a histogram for the data.

This visual summary shows that the distribution is skewed to the right – most students make few visits to a medical doctor, but there is a long 'tail'

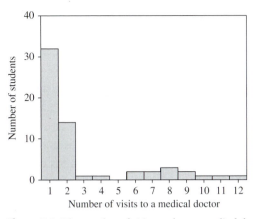

Figure 3.1 The number of visits made to a medical doctor during the past six months for 60 students chosen at random from a first-year biostatistics class of 600.

(and perhaps even a separate group) who have made six or more visits. Incidentally, looking at the graph you may be a little suspicious, since every student made at least one visit. When the class was asked about this, it was found that every student was required to undergo a routine medical examination during their first year at university, so these data are somewhat misleading in terms of indicating the health of the group.

You may be tempted to draw a line joining the midpoints of the tops of each bar to indicate the shape of the distribution, but this implies that the data on the X axis are continuous, which is not the case since visits are discrete whole numbers.

3.3.2   Frequency polygons or line graphs

If the data are continuous it is appropriate to draw a line linking the midpoint of the tops of each bar in a histogram. Here is an example for some continuous data that can be summarised as a histogram or as a frequency polygon (often called a line graph).

The time a person takes to respond to a stimulus is called their reaction time. This can be easily measured in the laboratory by getting them to press a button as soon as they see a light flash. The time elapsing between the instant of the flash and when the button is pressed is defined as the reaction time. A researcher suspected that an abnormally long reaction time might be a useful way of making an early diagnosis of certain neurological diseases, so they chose a group of 30 students at random from a first year biomedical science class and measured their reaction times in seconds. These data are shown below. Here too, nothing is very obvious from this list:

0.70, 0.50, 1.20, 0.80, 0.30, 0.34, 0.56, 0.41, 0.30, 1.20, 0.40, 0.64, 0.52, 0.38, 0.62, 0.47, 0.24, 0.55, 0.57, 0.61, 0.39, 0.55, 0.49, 0.41, 0.72, 0.71, 0.68, 0.49, 1.10, 0.59

First, since the data are continuous, they are not as easy to summarise as the discrete data in Figure 3.1. To display a histogram for continuous data you need to subdivide the data into the frequency of cases within a series of intervals of equal width. First you need to look at the range of the data (here reaction time varies from a minimum of 0.24 through to a maximum of 1.20 seconds) and decide on an interval width that will give you an informative display of the data. Here the chosen width is 0.999. Therefore, starting from 0.20, this will give 11 intervals, the first of which is 0.20–0.29. The chosen interval width needs to be one that shows the shape of the distribution. There would be no point in choosing a width that included all the data in just two intervals because you would only have two bars on the histogram. Nor would there be any point in choosing more than 20 intervals because this would give a lot of bars containing only a few data, which would be unlikely to reveal the shape of the distribution.

Once you have decided on an appropriate interval size, you need to count the number of students with a response time that falls within each (Table 3.1) and plot these frequencies on the Y axis against the intervals (indicated by the midpoint of each interval) on the X axis. This has been done in Figure 3.2(a). Finally, the midpoints of the tops of each rectangle have been joined by a line to give a frequency polygon, or line graph (Figure 3.2(b)).

Most students have short reaction times, but there is a distinct group of three who took a relatively long time to respond and who may be of further interest to the researcher.

3.3.3   Cumulative graphs

Often it is useful to display data as a histogram of cumulative frequencies. This is a graph that displays the progressive total of cases (starting at zero or zero per cent and finishing at the sample size or 100%) on the Y axis against

Table 3.1. Summary of the data for the reaction times in seconds of 30 students chosen at random from a first year biomedical class

Interval range	Number of students
0.20–0.29	1
0.30–0.39	5
0.40–0.49	6
0.50–0.59	7
0.60–0.69	4
0.70–0.79	3
0.80–0.89	1
0.90–0.99	0
1.00–1.09	0
1.10–1.19	1
1.20–1.29	2

Table 3.2. Summary of the data for the reaction time in seconds of 30 students chosen at random from a first year biomedical class as frequencies and cumulative frequencies

Interval range	Number of students	Cumulative frequency Total	Cumulative frequency Per cent
0.20–0.29	1	1	3.3
0.30–0.39	5	6	20
0.40–0.49	6	12	40
0.50–0.59	7	19	63.3
0.60–0.69	4	23	76.6
0.70–0.79	3	26	86.6
0.80–0.89	1	27	90
0.90–0.99	0	27	90
1.00–1.09	0	27	90
1.10–1.19	1	28	93.3
1.20–1.29	2	30	100

the increasing value of the variable on the X axis. Table 3.2 gives an example, using the data in Table 3.1.

A cumulative frequency graph can never decrease. Figure 3.3 displays the data in Table 3.2 as a frequency histogram.

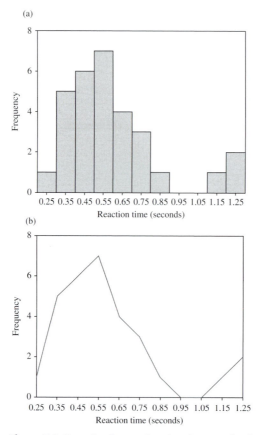

Figure 3.2 Data for the reaction time in seconds of 30 biomedical students selected at random, displayed as (a) a histogram and (b) a frequency polygon or line graph. The points on the frequency polygon (b) correspond to the midpoints of the bars on (a).

Although I have given the rather tedious manual procedures for constructing histograms, you will find that most statistical software packages have excellent graphics programs for displaying your data. These will automatically select an interval width, summarise the data, and plot the graph of your choice.

3.4   Displaying ordinal or nominal scale data

When you display data for nominal or ordinal scale variables you need to modify the form of the graph slightly because the categories are unlikely to

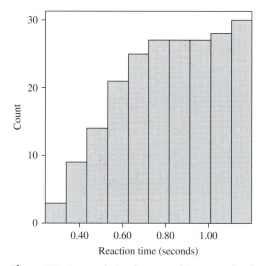

Figure 3.3 A cumulative frequency histogram for the reaction time of 30 students.

Table 3.3. The number of basal cell carcinomas detected and removed from eight locations on the body for 400 males aged from 40–50 years, during 12 months at a skin cancer clinic in Brisbane, Australia

Location	Number of basal cell carcinomas
Head (H)	211
Neck and shoulders (NS)	103
Arms (A)	74
Legs (L)	49
Upper back (UB)	94
Lower back (LB)	32
Chest (C)	21
Lower abdomen (LA)	12

be continuous, so the bars need to be separated to clearly indicate the lack of continuity. Here is an example for some nominal scale data. Table 3.3 gives the location of 596 basal cell carcinomas (a form of skin cancer that is most common on sun-exposed areas of the body) detected and removed

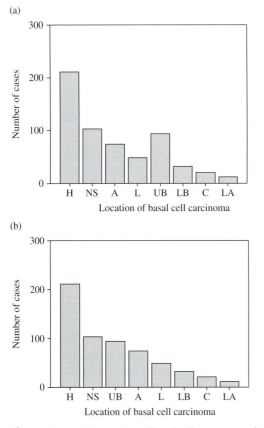

Figure 3.4 (a) The number of basal cell carcinomas detected and removed by location on the body during 12 months at a skin cancer clinic in Brisbane, Australia. (b) The same data but with the number of cases ranked in order from most to least.

from 400 males aged from 40 to 50 years treated during 12 months at a skin cancer clinic in Brisbane, Australia.

The locations have been defined as (a) head, (b) neck and shoulders, (c) arms, (d) legs, (e) upper back, (f) lower back, (g) chest, and (h) lower abdomen.

These can be displayed on a bar graph with the categories in any order along the X axis and the number of cases on the Y axis (Figure 3.4(a)). It often helps to rank the data in order of magnitude to aid interpretation (Figure 3.4(b)).

3.5   Bivariate data

Data where two variables have been measured on each experimental unit can often reveal patterns that may either suggest hypotheses, or be useful for testing them. Table 3.4 gives two lists of bivariate data for the number of dental caries (these are the holes that develop in decaying teeth) and the ages for 20 children between the ages of one and nine years from each of the cities of Uxford and Hambridge.

Looking at these data, there is not anything that stands out apart from an increase in the number of caries with age. If you calculate descriptive statistics such as the average age and average number of dental caries for each of the two groups (Table 3.5), they are not very informative either. (You have probably calculated the average for a set of data and this

Table 3.4. The number of dental caries and age of 20 children chosen at random from each of the two cities of Uxford and Hambridge

Uxford		Hambridge	
Caries	*Age*	*Caries*	*Age*
1	3	10	9
1	2	1	5
4	4	12	9
4	3	1	2
5	6	1	2
6	5	11	9
2	3	2	3
9	9	14	9
4	5	2	6
2	1	8	9
7	8	1	1
3	4	4	7
9	8	1	1
11	9	1	5
1	2	7	8
1	4	1	7
3	7	1	6
1	1	1	4
1	1	2	6
6	5	1	2

Table 3.5. The average number of dental caries and age of 20 children chosen at random from each of the two cities of Uxford and Hambridge

Uxford		Hambridge	
Caries	*Age*	*Caries*	*Age*
4.05	4.5 years	4.1	5.5 years

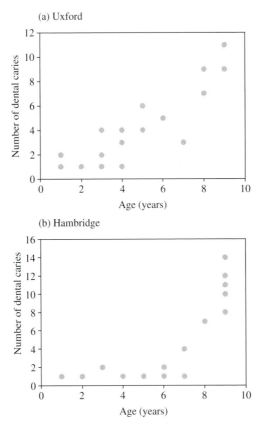

Figure 3.5 The number of dental caries plotted against the age of 20 children chosen at random from each of the two cities of (a) Uxford and (b) Hambridge.

procedure will be described in Chapter 6, but the average is the sum of all the values divided by the sample size.)

Table 3.5 shows that the sample from Hambridge had slightly more dental caries on average than the one from Uxford, but this is not surprising since the Hambridge sample was an average of one year older. If, however, you graph these data, patterns emerge. One way of displaying bivariate data is as a two-dimensional plot with increasing values of one variable on the horizontal (or X axis) and increasing values of the second variable on the vertical (or Y axis). Figure 3.5 shows both sets of data, with tooth decay (Y axis) plotted against child age (X axis) for each city.

These graphs show that tooth decay increases with age, but the pattern differs between cities – in Uxford the increase is fairly steady, but in Hambridge it remains low in children up to age seven but then suddenly increases. This might suggest hypotheses about the reasons why, or stimulate further investigation (perhaps a child dental care program, or water fluoridation, has been in place in Hambridge for the past eight years compared with no action on decay in Uxford). Of course, there is always the possibility that the samples are different due to chance, so perhaps the first step in any further investigation would be to repeat the sampling using much larger numbers of children from each city.

Graphs of this type are frequently used and you will have seen them many times before in newspapers, reports, scientific articles, and on television.

3.6   Multivariate data

Often life scientists have data for three or more variables measured on the same experimental unit. For example, a biomedical scientist might have data for age, blood pressure, and serum cholesterol for each individual in a sample of 20 people, or a marine ecologist might have data for the numbers of several species of marine invertebrates present in samples from a polluted area.

Results for three variables could be shown as three-dimensional graphs, but direct display is difficult for more than this number of variables. Some relatively new statistical techniques have made it possible to condense and summarise multivariate data in a two-dimensional display, but they are beyond the scope of this book.

3.7   Summary and conclusion

Graphs may reveal patterns in data sets that are not obvious from looking at lists or calculating descriptive statistics. Graphs can also provide an easily understood visual summary of a set of results. In later chapters there will be discussion of data displays such as boxplots and probability plots, which can be used to decide whether the data set is suitable for a particular analysis. Most modern statistical software packages have easy-to-use graphics options that produce high-quality graphs and figures. These packages are very useful for life scientists who are writing assignments, reports, or scientific publications.

4 | Introductory concepts of experimental design

4.1   Introduction

To generate hypotheses you often sample different groups or places (which is sometimes called a **mensurative** experiment because you usually measure something, such as height or weight, on each experimental unit) and explore these data for patterns or associations. To test hypotheses you may do mensurative experiments, or **manipulative** experiments where you change a condition and observe the effect of that change upon each experimental unit (like the experiment with millipedes and light described in Chapter 2). Often you may do several experiments of both types to test a particular hypothesis. The quality of your sampling and the design of your experiment can have an effect upon the outcome and determine whether your hypothesis is rejected or not. Therefore it is important to have an appropriate and properly designed experiment.

First, you should attempt to make your measurements as **accurate** and **precise** as possible so they are the best estimates of actual values.

Accuracy is the closeness of a measured value to the true value.
Precision is the 'spread' or variability of repeated measures of the same value.

For example, a thermometer that consistently gives a reading corresponding to a true temperature (e.g. 20°C) is both accurate and precise. Another that gives a reading consistently higher (e.g. +10°C) than a true temperature is not accurate, but it is very precise. In contrast, a thermometer that gives a fluctuating reading within a wide range of values around a true temperature is not precise and will usually be inaccurate except when the reading occasionally happens to correspond to the true temperature.

Inaccurate and imprecise measurements or a poor or unrealistic sampling design can result in the generation of inappropriate hypotheses. Measurement errors or a poor experimental design can give a false or misleading outcome that may result in the incorrect retention or rejection of an hypothesis.

The following is a discussion of some important essentials of sampling and experimental design.

4.2   Sampling – mensurative experiments

Mensurative experiments are often a good way of generating hypotheses or testing predictions from them. (An example of the latter is, 'I think millipedes are attracted to light at night. So if I sample 500 well-lit houses and 500 that are not well lit, the first group should, on average, contain more millipedes than the second.') You have to be careful when interpreting the results of mensurative experiments because you are sampling an **existing condition**, rather than **manipulating** conditions experimentally. There may be some other difference between your groups (e.g. well-lit houses may have a more 'open plan' design, which makes it easier for millipedes to get inside, and light may not be important at all).

4.2.1   Confusing a correlation with causality

A correlation between two variables means they vary together. A positive correlation means that high values of one variable are associated with high values of the other, while a negative correlation means that high values of one variable are associated with low values of the other. For example, the graph in Figure 4.1 shows a positive correlation between the population density of mice per square metre and the weight of wheat plants in kilograms per square metre from different parts of a large field.

Unfortunately a correlation is often mistakenly interpreted as indicating causality. It seems plausible that the amount of wheat might be the cause of differences in the numbers of mice (which may be eating the wheat or using it for shelter), but even if there is a very obvious correlation between any two variables it does not necessarily show that one is responsible for the other. The correlation may have occurred by chance, or a third unmeasured factor might determine the numbers of the two variables studied

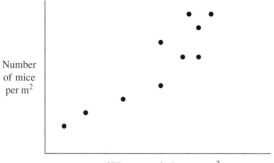

Figure 4.1 Example of a positive correlation between the numbers of mice and the weight of wheat plants per square metre.

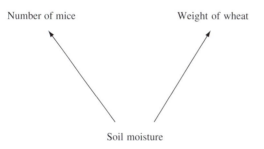

Figure 4.2 The involvement of a third variable 'Soil moisture' that determines the 'Number of mice' and 'Kilograms of wheat' per square metre. Even though there is no causal relationship between the number of mice and weight of wheat, the two variables are positively correlated.

(Figure 4.2). For example, soil moisture may determine both the number of mice and the weight of wheat. Therefore, although there is a causal relationship between soil moisture and each of the two variables, they are not causally related themselves.

4.2.2   The inadvertent inclusion of a third variable: sampling confounded in time

Occasionally researchers have no choice but to sample different populations of the same species, or different habitats, at different times. These results should be interpreted with great caution, since changes occurring over time may contribute to differences (or the lack of them) among samples. The sampling is said to be **confounded** in that more than one variable may be having an effect on the results. Here is an example.

An ecologist hypothesised that the density of above-ground vegetation might affect the population density of earthworms, and therefore sampled several different areas for these two variables. The work was very time consuming because the earthworms had to be sampled by taking cores of soil and unfortunately the ecologist had no help. Therefore, areas of low vegetation density were sampled in January, low to moderate density in February, moderate density in March, and high density in April. The sampling showed a negative correlation between vegetation density and earthworm density. Unfortunately, however, the density of earthworms was the same in all areas, but decreased as the year progressed (and the ecologist did not know this). Therefore, the negative correlation between earthworm density and vegetation density was an artefact of the sampling of different places being confounded in time. This is an example of a common problem, and you are likely to find similar cases in many published scientific papers and reports.

4.2.3   The need for independent samples in mensurative experiments

Frequently researchers sample the numbers, or population density, of a species in relation to an environmental gradient (such as depth in a lake), to see if there is any correlation between density of the species and the gradient of interest.

There is an obvious need to **replicate** the sampling – that is, to independently estimate density more than once. For example, consider sampling Dark Lake, Wisconsin, to investigate the population density of freshwater prawns in relation to depth.

If you only sampled at one place (Figure 4.3(a)) the results would not be a good indication of changes in the population density of prawns with depth in the lake. The sampling needs to be replicated, but there is little value in repeatedly sampling one small area (e.g. by taking several samples under '****' in Figure 4.3(b)) since this still will not give an accurate indication of changes in population density with depth across the whole lake (although it may give a very accurate indication of conditions in that particular part of the lake). This sort of sampling is one aspect of what Hurlbert (1984) called

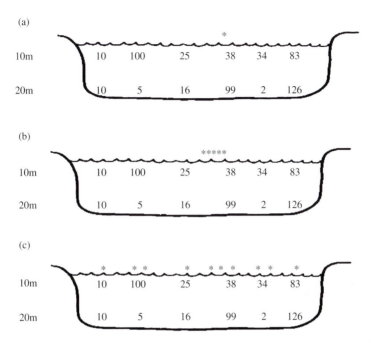

Figure 4.3 Variation in the number of freshwater prawns per cubic metre of water at two different depths (10 m and 20 m) in Dark Lake, Wisconsin. (a) An unreplicated sample taken at only one place (*) would give a very misleading indication of changes in the population density of prawns with depth within the entire lake. (b) Several replicates taken at only one place (*****) would still give a very misleading indication of conditions within the entire lake. (c) Several replicates taken at random across the lake would give a better indication within the entire lake.

pseudoreplication, which is still a very common flaw in a lot of scientific research. The replicates are 'pseudo' – sham or unreal – because they are unlikely to truly describe what is occurring across the entire area being discussed (in this case the lake). A better design would be to sample at several places chosen at random within the lake as shown in Figure 4.3(c).

This type of inappropriate sampling is very common. Here is another example. A researcher sampled a large coral reef by dropping a 1 m² square frame, subdivided into a grid of 100 equal-sized squares, at random in one place only and then took one sample from each of these smaller squares. Although these 100 replicates may very accurately describe conditions within the sampling frame they may not necessarily describe the remaining 9999 m² of the reef and would be pseudoreplicates if the results were interpreted in this way. A more appropriate design would be to sample 100 replicates chosen at random across the whole reef.

4.2.4 The need to repeat the sampling on several occasions and elsewhere

In the example described above, the results of sampling Dark Lake can only confidently be discussed in relation to that particular lake on that day. Therefore, when interpreting results you need to be cautious. Sampling the same lake on several different occasions will strengthen the findings, and may be sufficient if you are only interested in that lake. Sampling more than one lake will make the results more able to be generalised. Inappropriate generalisation is another example of pseudoreplication since data from one location may not hold in the more general case. At the same time, however, even if your study is limited you can still make more general predictions from your findings provided these are clearly identified as predictions.

4.3 Manipulative experiments

4.3.1 Independent replicates

It is essential to have several independent replicates of any treatment used in an experiment. I mentioned this briefly when describing the millipedes and light experiment in Chapter 2 and said if there were only one lit and one unlit tile any difference between them could have simply been due to chance or some other unknown factor(s). As the number of randomly chosen independent replicates increases, so does the likelihood that any difference between the experimental group and the control group is a result of the experimental treatment. The following example is deliberately absurd because I will use it later in this chapter to discuss a lack of replication that is not so obvious.

Imagine you were asked to test the hypothesis that vitamin C caused guinea pigs to grow more rapidly. You obtained two six-week-old guinea pigs of the same sex and weight, caged them separately, and offered one an unlimited amount of commercial rodent food plus 20 mg of vitamin C per day, while the other guinea pig was only offered an unlimited amount of commercial rodent food. The guinea pigs were re-weighed after three months and the results were obvious – the guinea pig that received vitamin C was 40% heavier than the one that had not.

This result is consistent with the hypothesis but there is an obvious flaw in the experiment – with only one guinea pig in each treatment, any differences between treatments may be due to differences between the guinea pigs, differences between the treatment cages, or both. (For example, the slow-growing guinea pig may, by chance, have been heavily infested with intestinal parasites). There is a need to replicate this experiment and the replicates need to be truly independent – for example it is not sufficient to have ten 'vitamin C' guinea pigs together in one cage and ten control guinea pigs in another, because any differences between treatments may still be caused by some difference between the cages. There will be more about this shortly.

4.3.2   Control treatments

Control treatments are needed because they allow the experimenter to isolate the reason why something is occurring in an experiment by comparing two treatments that differ by only **one factor**. Frequently the need for a rigorous experimental design makes it necessary to have several different treatments, more than one of which can be considered controls.

Here is an example. Herbivorous species of marine snails are often common in rock pools on the shore, where they eat algae that grow on the sides of the pools. Very occasionally these snails are seen being attacked and eaten by carnivorous species of intertidal snails, which also occur in the rock pools. An ecologist was surprised that such attacks occurred so infrequently and hypothesised that this was because the herbivorous snails showed 'avoidance' by climbing out of the water in response to water borne odours from their predators.

The null hypothesis is, 'herbivorous snails will not avoid their predators' and the alternate hypothesis is, 'herbivorous snails will avoid their predators'. One prediction that might distinguish between these hypotheses is that, 'herbivorous snails will crawl out of their pool when a predatory snail is added'. This could be tested by dropping a predatory snail into a rock pool where some herbivorous snails are present and seeing how many crawled out during the next five minutes.

Unfortunately, this experiment is not controlled. By adding a predator and waiting for five minutes, several things have happened to the

Table 4.1. Breakdown of three treatments into their effects upon herbivorous snails

Predator	Control for disturbance	Control for time
predator disturbance time	disturbance time	time

herbivorous snails in the pool. Certainly, you are adding a predator. But the pool is also being **disturbed**, simply by adding something (the predator) to it. Also, the experiment is not well controlled in terms of **time**, since five minutes have elapsed while the experiment is being done. Therefore, even if all the herbivorous snails crawled out of the pool, the experimenter could not confidently attribute this to the addition of the predator – the snails may have crawled out in response to disturbance, because the pool had warmed up in the sun, or many other reasons.

One improvement to this experiment would be a control for the disturbance associated with adding a predator. A popular treatment to control for this is to include another pool into which a small stone about the size of the predator is dropped, as 'something added to the pool'. Another important improvement would include a control pool to which nothing was added.

At this stage, by incorporating the improvements, you would have three treatments. Table 4.1 lists what these treatments are doing to the snails.

For such a simple hypothesis, 'herbivorous snails will avoid their predators', the experiment has already expanded to three treatments. But many ecologists are likely to say that even this design is not adequate, since the 'predator' treatment **is the only one in which a snail has been added to a pool.** Therefore, even if the snails all crawled out of the pools in the treatment to which the predator had been added but remained submerged in the other two treatments, the response may have been only a response to the addition of **any** living snail, rather than a predator. Ideally, a fourth treatment should be included, where an herbivorous snail is added, to control for this (Table 4.2).

You may, at this point, be thinking that the above design is far too finicky. Nevertheless, experiments have to have appropriate controls so

Table 4.2. Breakdown of four treatments into their effects upon herbivorous snails

Predator	Control for snail	Control for disturbance	Control for time
predator	herbivore		
disturbance	disturbance	disturbance	
time	time	time	time

that the effects of each potentially contributing factor can be isolated. Furthermore, the design would have to include replicates as well – you could not just do it once, using four pools, since any difference among treatments may result from some difference among the pools rather than the actual treatments applied. I have done this experiment (McKillup and McKillup, 1993) and included all the treatments listed in Table 4.2 with six replicates, using 30 pools altogether.

It is often difficult to work out what control treatments you need to incorporate in a manipulative experiment. One way to clarify these is to list all of the things you are actually doing to an experimental treatment and make sure you have appropriate controls for each.

4.3.3   Other common types of manipulative experiments where treatments are confounded with time

Many experiments confound treatments with time. For example, experiments designed to evaluate the effects of drugs often measure some physiological variable (e.g. blood pressure) of the same group of experimental subjects before and after a treatment. Any change is attributed to the effect of the drug.

Here, however, several different things have been done to the treatment group. I will use blood pressure as an example, but they apply to any 'before and after' experiment.

First, time has elapsed, and blood pressure can change over a matter of minutes or hours in response to many factors, even room temperature.

Second, the group has been given a drug, but studies have shown that administration of even an empty capsule or an injection of saline (these are called **placebo** treatments) can affect a person's blood pressure.

Third, each person in the group has had their blood pressure measured twice. Many people are 'white coat hypertensive' – their blood pressure increases substantially at the sight of a physician approaching with the inflatable cuff and pressure gauge used to measure blood pressure.

An improvement to this experiment could include a group that was treated in exactly the same way as the experimental group, except that the subjects were given an appropriate placebo. This would at least isolate the effect of the drug from the other ways in which both groups had been disturbed. Consequently, well-designed medical experiments often include 'sham operations' where the control subjects are operated on in the same way as the experimental subjects, except that they do not receive the experimental manipulation. For example, early experiments to investigate the function of the parathyroid glands, which are small patches of tissue present within the thyroid, included an experimental treatment where the parathyroids were completely removed from several dogs, while a control group of dogs had their thyroids exposed and cut, but the parathyroids were left in place.

4.3.4   Pseudoreplication

One of the nastiest pitfalls is appearing to have a replicated manipulative experimental design, which really is not replicated. This is another aspect of 'pseudoreplication' described by Hurlbert (1984) who invented the word – before then it was just called 'bad design'. Here is an example that relates back to the discussion about the need for replicates.

An aquacultural scientist hypothesised that a diet which included excess vitamin A would increase the growth rate of prawns. They were aware of the need to replicate their experiment, so they set up two treatment ponds, each containing 1000 prawns of the same species and of similar weight and age from the same hatchery. One pond was chosen at random and the 1000 prawns within it fed commercial prawn food plus vitamin A, while the 1000 prawns in the second pond were only fed commercial prawn food. After six months the prawns were harvested and weighed. The prawns that received vitamin A were twice as heavy, on average, as the ones that had not. The scientist was delighted – an experiment with 1000 replicates of each treatment had produced a result consistent with the hypothesis.

Unfortunately, there are **not** 1000 truly independent replicates in each pond. All prawns receiving vitamin A were in pond 1 and all those receiving only standard food were in pond 2. Therefore, any difference in growth may, or may not, have been due to the vitamin – it could equally well have been due to some other (perhaps unknown) difference between the two ponds. The experimental replicates are the ponds, not the prawns, so the experiment has no effective replication at all and is essentially the same as the absurd unreplicated guinea pig experiment described earlier in this chapter.

An improvement to the design would be to run each treatment in several ponds. For example, an experiment with five ponds in each treatment, each containing 200 prawns, has at least been replicated five times. But here too, it is still necessary to have truly independent replicates – you can not subdivide two ponds into five enclosures and run one treatment in each pond. This is one case of **apparent replication**, and here are four examples.

1 Even if you have several separate replicates of each treatment (say five treatment aquaria and five control aquaria), the arrangement of these can lead to a lack of independence. First you may have your treatment aquaria all clumped together at one end of a laboratory bench and the experimental aquaria at the other. But there may be some known or unknown feature of the laboratory (e.g. light levels, ventilation, disturbance) that affects one group of aquaria differently to the other (Figure 4.4(a)).

2 Replicates placed alternately. If you decided to get around the clustering problem by placing treatments and controls alternately (i.e. by placing, from left to right, treatment 1, control 1; treatment 2, control 2; treatment 3 etc. . . .), there can still be problems. Just by chance all the treatment aquaria (or all the controls) might be under regularly placed laboratory ceiling lights, next to windows, or subject to some other regular feature you are not even aware of (Figure 4.4(b)).

3 Often, because of a shortage of equipment, you may have to have all of your replicates of one temperature treatment in only one controlled temperature cabinet, and all replicates of another temperature in only one other. Unfortunately, if there is something peculiar to one cabinet, in addition to temperature, then either the experimental or control treatment may be affected. This pattern is called 'isolative segregation' (Figure 4.4(c)).

4 The final example is more subtle. Imagine you decided to test the hypothesis that, 'Water with a high nitrogen content increases the

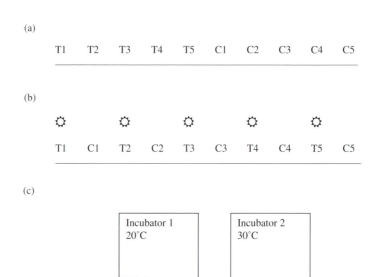

Figure 4.4 Three cases of apparent pseudoreplication. (a) Clustering of replicates means that there is no independence among controls or treatments. (b) A regular arrangement of treatments and controls may, by chance, correspond to some feature of the environment (here the very obvious ceiling lights) that might affect the results. (c) Clustering of temperature treatments within particular incubators.

growth of freshwater mussels.' You set up five control aquaria and five experimental aquaria, which were placed on the bench in a completely randomised pattern, to get around examples 1 and 2 above. All tanks had to have water constantly flowing through them, so you set up one storage tank containing water high in nitrogen and one containing water low in nitrogen. Water from each storage tank was piped into five aquaria as shown in Figure 4.5.

This looks fine, but unfortunately all of the five aquaria within each treatment are sharing the same water. All in the 'high nitrogen' treatment receive water high in nitrogen from Tank A and all aquaria in the control receive water low in nitrogen from Tank B, so any difference in mussel growth between treatments may be due either to the nitrogen or some other feature of the storage tanks. Really, therefore, this design is little better than the case of isolative segregation (example 3 above). Ideally, each aquarium should have its own separate and independent supply. Finally, the allocation of replicate tanks to treatments should be done

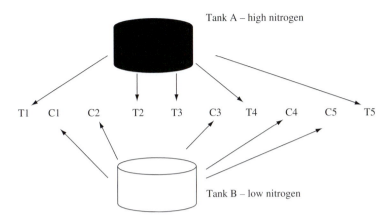

Figure 4.5 The positions of the treatment tanks are randomised, but all tanks within a treatment share water from one supply tank.

using a method that removes any possibility of unintentional bias by the experimenter. (For example, the toss of a coin was used to allocate pairs of tiles to lit and unlit treatments in the experiment with millipedes and light described in Section 2.2.)

4.4   Sometimes you can only do an unreplicated experiment

Although replication is desirable in any experiment, there are some cases where it is not possible. For example, when doing large-scale mensurative or manipulative experiments on systems such as lakes or rivers there may be only one polluted lake or river available to study. Although you cannot attribute the reason for any difference, or the lack of it, to the treatment (e.g. a polluted versus a relatively unpolluted river), since you only have one replicate, the results are still useful. First, they are still evidence for or against your hypothesis and can be cautiously discussed in the light of the lack of replication. Second, it may be possible to achieve replication by analysing your results in conjunction with those from similar studies done elsewhere by other researchers. This is called a **meta-analysis**. Finally, the results of a large-scale but unreplicated experiment may suggest smaller-scale experiments that can be done with replication so that you can continue to test the hypothesis.

4.5   Realism

Even an apparently well-designed mensurative or manipulative experiment may still suffer from a lack of realism. Here are two examples.

The first is a mensurative experiment on the incidence of testicular torsion. Testicular torsion can occur in males when the testicular artery supplying the testis with oxygenated blood becomes twisted. This can restrict or cut off the blood supply and thereby damage or kill the testis. Apparently this is an extremely painful condition and usually requires surgery to either restore blood flow or remove the damaged testis. Since the testes retract closer to the body as temperature decreases, a physician hypothesised that the likelihood of torsion would be greater during winter compared with summer. Their alternate hypothesis was, 'Retraction of the testis during cold weather increases the incidence of testicular torsion.' The null hypothesis was, 'Retraction of the testis during cold weather does not increase the incidence of testicular torsion.'

The physician found that the incidence of testicular torsion was twice as high during winter compared with summer in a small town in Alaska. Unfortunately there were very few affected males (six altogether) in the sample, so this difference may have occurred simply by chance, making it impossible to distinguish between these hypotheses. Later, another researcher obtained data from a much larger sample of 96 affected males from hospital records in north Queensland, Australia. They found no difference in the incidence of testicular torsion between summer and winter, but this may not have been a realistic test of the hypothesis, because even Alaskan summers are considerably colder than north Queensland winters.

Second, an experiment to investigate factors affecting the selection of breeding sites by the mosquito *Anopheles farauti* offered adult females a choice of salinities ranging from 0, 5, 10, 15, 20, 25, 30, and 35 parts per thousand. Eggs were laid in all but the two highest salinities (30 and 35 parts per thousand). The conclusion was that salinity significantly affects the choice of breeding sites by mosquitoes. Unfortunately the salinity in the habitat where the mosquitoes occurred never exceeded ten parts per thousand, again making the choice of treatments unrealistic.

4.6   A bit of common sense

By now, you may be quite daunted by the challenge of being able to design a good experiment. Provided, however, that you have appropriate controls, replicates, and have also thought about any obvious problems of pseudoreplication and realism, you are well on the way to a good design. Furthermore, the desire for a near-perfect design has to be balanced against financial constraints as well as space and time available to do the experiment. Often it is not possible to have more than two incubators, or as many replicates as you would like. It also depends on the type of life science you do. For example, many microbiologists working with organisms they grow on agar plates, where conditions can be strictly controlled, would never be concerned about clustering of replicates or isolative segregation because they were confident that conditions did not vary in different parts of their laboratory and their incubators only differed in relation to temperature. Most of the time they may be right, but considerations about experimental design need to be borne in mind by all life scientists.

Also, you may not have the resources to do a large manipulative field experiment at more than one site. Although, strictly speaking, the results cannot be generalised to other sites, they may nevertheless apply, and careful interpretation and discussion of results can make more general predictions. For example, the 'millipede and light' experiment described in Chapter 2 was initially done during one night at one site. It was repeated on the following night at the same site in the presence of some colleagues (who were initially rather sceptical), and later at two other sites, as well as in the laboratory. All the results were consistent with the hypothesis, so I concluded, 'Portuguese millipedes are attracted to visible light at night.' Nevertheless, the hypothesis may not be correct or apply to all populations of *O. moreleti*, but, to date, there has been no evidence to the contrary.

4.7   Designing a 'good' experiment

Designing a well-controlled, appropriately replicated and realistic experiment has been described by some researchers as an 'art'. It is not, but there are often several different ways to test the same hypothesis, and hence several different experiments that could be done. Consequently, it is

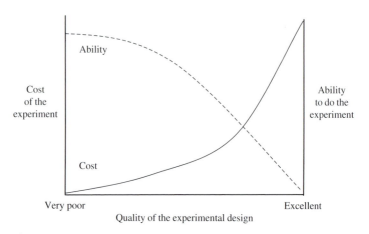

Figure 4.6 An example of the trade off between the cost and ability to do an experiment. As the quality of the experimental design increases, so does the cost of the experiment (solid line), while the ability to do the experiment decreases (dashed line). Your design usually has to be a compromise between one that is practicable, affordable, and of sufficient rigour.

difficult to set a guide to designing experiments beyond an awareness of the general principles discussed in this chapter.

4.7.1 Good design versus the ability to do the experiment

It has often been said, 'There is no such thing as a perfect experiment.' One inherent problem is that, as a design gets better and better, the cost in time and equipment also increases, but the ability to actually do the experiment decreases (Figure 4.6). An absolutely perfect design may be impossible to carry out. Therefore, every researcher must choose a design that is 'good enough' but still practical. There are no rules for this – the decision on design is in the hands of the researcher, and will be eventually judged by their colleagues who examine any report from the work.

4.8   Conclusion

The above discussion only superficially covers some important aspects of experimental design. Considering how easy it is to make a mistake, you probably will not be surprised that a lot of published scientific papers have serious flaws in design or interpretation that could have been avoided.

Work with major problems in the design of experiments is still being done and, quite alarmingly, many researchers are not aware of these. As an example, after teaching the material in this chapter I often ask my students to find a published paper, review and criticise the experimental design, and then offer constructive suggestions for improvement. Many have later reported that it was far easier to find a flawed paper than they expected.

5 | Probability helps you make a decision about your results

5.1   Introduction

Most science is comparative. Researchers often need to know if a particular experimental treatment has had an effect, or if there are differences among a particular variable measured at several different locations. For example, does a new drug affect blood pressure, does a diet high in vitamin C reduce the risk of liver cancer in humans, or is there a relationship between vegetation cover and the population density of rabbits? But when you make these sorts of comparisons, any differences among treatments or among areas sampled may be real or they may simply be the sort of variation that occurs by chance among samples from the same population.

Here is an example using blood pressure. A biomedical scientist was interested in seeing if the newly synthesised drug 'Arterolin B' had any effect on blood pressure in humans. A group of six humans had their systolic blood pressure measured before and after administration of a dose of Arterolin B. The average systolic blood pressure was 118.33 mm Hg before and 128.83 mm Hg after being given the drug (Table 5.1).

The average change in blood pressure from before to after administration of the drug is quite large (an increase of 10.5 mm Hg), but by looking at the data you can see there is a lot of variation among individuals – blood pressure went up in three cases, down in two, and stayed the same for the remaining person.

Even so, the scientist might conclude that a dose of Arterolin B increases blood pressure. But there is a problem (apart from the poor experimental design that has no controls for time or the disturbing effect of having one's blood pressure measured). How do you know that the effect of the drug is **meaningful** or **significant?** Perhaps this change occurred by chance and the drug had no effect. Somehow you need a way of helping you **make a**

Table 5.1. The systolic blood pressure in mm Hg for six people before and after being given the experimental drug Arterolin B

Person	Before	After
1	100	108
2	120	120
3	120	150
4	140	135
5	80	120
6	150	140
Average	118.33	128.83

decision about your results. This led to the development of statistical tests and a commonly agreed upon level of statistical significance.

5.2   Statistical tests and significance levels

Statistical tests are just a way of working out **the probability of obtaining the observed, or an even more extreme, difference among samples (or between an observed and expected value) if a specific hypothesis (usually the null of no difference) is true.** Once the probability is known, the experimenter can make a decision about the difference, using criteria that are uniformly used and understood. Here is a very easy example where the probability of every possible outcome can be calculated.

Imagine you have a large sack containing 5000 white and 5000 black beads that are otherwise identical. All of these beads are well mixed together. They are a population of 10 000 beads.

You take one bead out at random, without looking in the sack. Since there are equal numbers of black and white, your probability of getting a black one is 50%, or ½, which is also your chance of getting a white one. The chance of getting **either** a black or white bead is the sum of these probabilities: (½ + ½) which is 1.0 (or 100%) since there are no other colours. (If you are unsure about probability, there is a short explanation of the concepts you will need for this book in Box 5.1.)

Now consider what happens if you take out a sample of six beads in sequence, one after the other, without looking in the sack. Each bead is

Box 5.1 Basic concepts of probability

The probability of any event can only vary between 0 and 1 (which correspond to 0 and 100%). If an event is certain to occur, it has a probability of 1; while, if it is certain the event will **not** occur, it has a probability of 0.

The probability of a particular event is the number of outcomes giving that event, divided by the total number of possible outcomes. For example, when you toss a coin there are only two possible outcomes – a head or a tail. These two events are mutually exclusive – you cannot get both. Consequently, the probability of a head is 1 divided by $2 = ½$ (and thus the probability of a tail is also ½).

The addition rule

The probability of getting **either** a head **or** a tail is $½ + ½ = 1$. This is an example of the **addition rule**: when several outcomes are mutually exclusive, the probability of getting any of these is the sum of their separate probabilities. (Therefore, the probability of getting either a 1, 2, 3, or 4 when rolling a six-sided die is 4/6.)

The multiplication rule

Independent events. To calculate the joint probability of two or more independent events (for example, a head followed by another head in two independent tosses of a coin) you simply multiply the independent probabilities together. Therefore, the probability of getting two heads with two tosses of a coin are $½ × ½ = ¼$. The chance of a head **or** a tail with two tosses is ½, because there are two ways of obtaining this: HT or TH.

Related events. If the events are not independent (for example, the first event being a number in the range of 1–3 inclusive when rolling a six-sided die and the second event being that this is an even number), the multiplication rule also applies, but you have to multiply the probability of one event by the **conditional probability** of the second.

When rolling a die the independent probability of a number from 1 to 3 is $3/6 = ½$, and the independent probability of any even number is also ½ (the even numbers are 2, 4, or 6 divided by the six possible outcomes).

If, however, you have already rolled a number from 1 to 3, the probability of that restricted set of outcomes being an even number is 1/3 (because '2' is the only even number possible in this set of three outcomes). Therefore, the probability of **both** related events is $\frac{1}{2} \times 1/3 = 1/6$. You can look at this the other way – the chance of an even number when rolling a die is $\frac{1}{2}$ (you would get numbers 2, 4, or 6) and the probability of one of these numbers being in the range from 1 to 3 is 1/3 (the number 2 out of these three outcomes). Therefore the probability of both is again $\frac{1}{2} \times 1/3 = 1/6$.

replaced after it is drawn and the contents of the sack remixed before taking out the next, so these are independent events.

Here are all of the possible outcomes. You may get six black beads or six white ones (both outcomes are very unlikely); five black and one white, or one black and five white (which is more likely); four black and two white, or two black and four white (which is even more likely); or three black and three white (which is very likely because the proportion of beads in the sack is 1:1).

The probability of getting six black beads in sequence is the probability of getting one black one ($\frac{1}{2}$) multiplied by itself six times, which is $\frac{1}{2} \times \frac{1}{2} \times \frac{1}{2} \times \frac{1}{2} \times \frac{1}{2} \times \frac{1}{2} = 1/64$.

The probability of getting six white beads is also 1/64.

The probability of five black and one white is greater because there are six ways of getting this combination (WBBBBB or BWBBBB or BBWBBB or BBBWBB or BBBBWB or BBBBBW) giving 6/64.

There is the same probability (6/64) of getting five white and one black.

The probability of four black and two white is even greater because there are 15 ways of getting this combination (WWBBBB, BWWBBB, BBWWBB, BBBWWB, BBBBWW, WBWBBB, WBBWBB, WBBBWB, WBBBBW, BWBWBB, BWBBWB, BWBBBW, BBWBWB, BBWBBW, BBBWBW) giving 15/64.

There is the same probability (15/64) of getting four white and two black.

Finally, the probability of three black and three white (there are 20 ways of getting this combination) is 20/64.

You can summarise all of the outcomes as a table of probabilities (Table 5.2).

These probabilities are shown as a histogram in Figure 5.1. Note that the distribution is symmetrical with a peak corresponding to the cases where half the beads will be black and half white. (Incidentally, this is

Table 5.2. The probabilities of obtaining all possible combinations of black and white beads in samples of six from a large population where there are equal numbers of black and white beads

Number of black	Number of white	Probability of this outcome	Percentage of cases likely to give this result
6	0	1/64	1.56
5	1	6/64	9.38
4	2	15/64	23.44
3	3	20/64	31.25
2	4	15/64	23.44
1	5	6/64	9.38
0	6	1/64	1.56
Total		64/64	100%

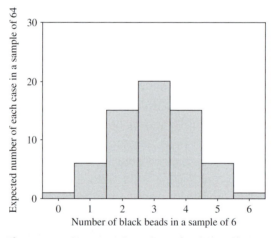

Figure 5.1 The expected numbers of each possible mixture of colours when drawing six beads independently with replacement on 64 different occasions from a large population containing 50% black and 50% white beads.

an example of the **binomial distribution,** which will be discussed in Chapter 17.)

Therefore, if you were given a sack containing 50% black and 50% white beads, from which you drew six, you would have a very high probability of drawing a sample that contains beads of both colours. It is very unlikely you would get only six black or six white (the probability of each is 1/64, so the probability of **either** six black or six white is the sum of these which is only 2/64, or 0.0313 or 3.13%).

5.3   What has this got to do with making a decision or statistical testing?

The statistician Sir Ronald Fisher proposed that, if the probability of getting this or a more extreme difference between the expected outcome (the null hypothesis discussed in Chapter 2) and the actual outcome is **less than 5%**, then it is appropriate to conclude that the difference is **statistically significant** (Fisher, 1954).

There is no biological reason for the choice of 5% (which is the same as 1/20 or 0.05). It is the probability that many researchers use as a standard 'statistical significant level'.

Using the example of the beads in the sack, if your null hypothesis specified that there were equal numbers of black and white beads in the population, you could do an experiment to test it by drawing out a sample of six beads as described above. If all six were black or all were white, the probability of either outcome (which in this case are the most extreme departures from the expected under the null hypothesis) is only 3.13% and would be considered statistically significant. A researcher would reject the null hypothesis and conclude that the sample did **not** come from a population containing equal numbers of black and white beads.

5.4   Making the wrong decision

If the proportions of black and white beads in the sack really were equal, then most of the time a sample of six beads would contain both colours. But, if the beads in the sample were all only black or all only white, a researcher would decide the sack (the population) did not contain 50% black and 50% white. Here they would have made the wrong decision, but this would not happen very often (the probability of either of these outcomes is 2/64).

The unavoidable problem with using probability to help you make a decision is that there is **always** a chance of making a wrong decision and you have no way of telling when you have done this.

As described above, if a researcher got a sample of six of one colour, they would decide that the population (the contents of the bag) was not 50% black and 50% white when really it was. This mistake, where the null hypothesis of equal numbers is inappropriately rejected, is called a **Type 1 error**.

There is another problem too. Sometimes an unknown population is different to the expected (e.g. it may contain 90% white beads and 10% black ones), but the sample taken (e.g. four white and two black) is not significantly different to the expected outcome predicted by the hypothesis of 50:50. In this case the researcher would decide the composition of the population was the one expected under the null hypothesis (50:50), even though it was not. This mistake, when the alternate hypothesis holds but is inappropriately rejected, is called a **Type 2 error**.

Every time you do a statistical test you run the risk of a Type 1 or Type 2 error. There will be more discussion of these errors in Chapter 8, but they are unavoidably associated with using probability to help you make a decision.

5.5   Other probability levels

Sometimes, depending on the hypothesis being tested, a researcher may decide that the 'less than 5%' significance level (with its 5% chance of inappropriately rejecting the null hypothesis) is too risky.

Here is a medical example. Malaria is caused by a parasitic protozoan that is carried by certain species of mosquito. When an infected mosquito bites a person the protozoans are injected into the person's bloodstream, where they reproduce inside red blood cells. A small proportion of malarial infections progress to cerebral malaria, where the parasite infects cells in the person's brain, causing severe inflammation and often death. A biomedical scientist was asked to test a new and extremely expensive drug that was hoped to reduce mortality in people suffering from cerebral malaria. A large experiment was done, where half of cerebral malaria cases chosen at random received the new drug and the other half did not. The survival of both groups over the next month was compared. The alternate hypothesis was, 'There will be increased survival of the drug-treated group compared to the control.'

Here, the prohibitive cost of the drug meant that the manufacturer had to be very confident that it was of real use before recommending and marketing it. Therefore, the risk of a Type 1 error (significantly greater survival in the experimental group compared with the control simply by chance) when using the 5% significance level might be considered too risky. Instead, the researcher might decide to reduce the risk of Type 1 error by using the 1% or even 0.1% level and only recommend the drug if the reduction in mortality was so marked that it was significant at these levels.

Here is an example of the opposite case. Before releasing any new pharmaceutical product on the market it has to be assessed for side effects. There were concerns that the new sunscreen 'Bayray Blockout 2020' might cause an increase in pimples among frequent users. A pharmaceutical scientist ran an experiment using 200 high-school students during their summer holiday. Each was asked to apply Bayray Blockout 2020 to their left cheek and the best-selling but boringly named 'Sensible Suncare' to their right cheek every morning, and then spend the next hour sunbathing. After six weeks the number of pimples per square cm on each cheek were counted and compared. The alternate hypothesis was, 'Bayray Blockout 2020 causes an increase in pimple numbers compared with Sensible Suncare.' Here, an increase could be disastrous for sales, so the scientist decided on a significance level of 10% rather than the conventional 5%. Even though there was a 10% chance (double the usual risk) of a Type 1 error, the company could not take the chance that Bayray Blockout 2020 increased the incidence of pimples.

The most commonly used significance level is 5%, which is 0.05. If you decide to use a different level in an analysis, the decision needs to be made, justified, and clearly specified before the experiment is done.

For a significant result the actual probability is also important. For example, a probability of 0.04 is not very much less than 0.05. In contrast, a probability of 0.002 is very much less than 0.05. Therefore, even though both are significant, the result with the lowest probability gives much stronger evidence for rejecting the null hypothesis.

5.6   How are probability values reported?

The symbol used for the chosen significance level (e.g. 0.05) is the Greek α (alpha). Often you will see the probability reported as $P < 0.05$ or $P < 0.01$ or $P < 0.001$. These mean, respectively, 'The probability is less than 0.05' or 'The probability is less than 0.01' or 'The probability is less than 0.001.'

N.S. means 'not significant,' which is when the probability is 0.05 or more ($P \geq 0.05$). Of course, as noted above, if you have specified a significance level of 0.05 and get a result with a probability of less than 0.001, this is far stronger evidence for your alternate hypothesis than a result with a probability of 0.04.

5.7   All statistical tests do the same basic thing

In the 'beads from a sack' example all of the possible outcomes were listed and the probability of each was calculated directly.

Some statistical tests do this. Most, however, use a formula to produce a number called a **statistic**. The probability of getting each possible value of the statistic has been previously calculated, so you can use the formula to get the numerical value of the statistic, look up the probability of that value in a published set of statistical tables, and make your decision to retain the null hypothesis if it has a probability of ≥ 0.05 or reject it if it has a probability of <0.05. Most statistical software packages now available will generate the probability as well as the statistic, so you do not even need a set of tables.

5.8   A very simple example – the chi-square test for goodness of fit

Here is an example to illustrate the concepts discussed above, using one of the simplest statistical tests.

The chi-square test for goodness of fit compares observed ratios with expected ratios for nominal scale data. Imagine you have done a genetics experiment on pelt colour in guinea pigs, where you expect a 3:1 ratio of brown to albino offspring. You have obtained 100 offspring altogether, so you would expect the numbers in the sample to be 75 brown to 25 albino, but you actually get 86 brown and 14 albino offspring. This difference from the expected frequencies might be due to chance, it may be because your null hypothesis is incorrect, or a combination of both. You need to decide whether this result is significantly different from the one expected under the null hypothesis.

This is the same as the concept developed in Section 5.2 when I discussed sampling a sack of beads, except that the chi-square test for goodness of fit generates a statistic (a number) that allows you to easily estimate the probability of the observed (or any greater) deviation from the expected outcome. It is so simple you can do it on a calculator.

To calculate the value of chi-square, which is symbolised by the Greek χ^2, you take each expected value away from its equivalent observed value, square the difference, and divide this by the expected value. These separate values (two in the case above) are added together to give the chi-square statistic.

First, here is the chi-square statistic for an expected ratio that is the same as the observed (observed numbers 75 brown : 25 albino; expected 75 brown : 25 albino). Therefore the two categories of data are 'brown' and 'albino':

$$\chi^2 = \frac{(75 - 75)^2}{75} + \frac{(25 - 25)^2}{25} = 0 + 0 = 0$$

The value of chi-square is zero when there is no difference between the observed and expected values.

As the difference between the observed and expected values increases, so does the value of chi-square. Here the observed ratio is 74 and 26 (the value of chi-square can only be a positive number because you always square the difference between the observed and expected values):

$$\chi^2 = \frac{(74 - 75)^2}{75} + \frac{(26 - 25)^2}{25} = 0.0533$$

For an observed ratio of 70:30, the chi-square statistic is:

$$\chi^2 = \frac{(70 - 75)^2}{75} + \frac{(30 - 25)^2}{25} = 1.333$$

When you take samples from a population in a 'category' experiment you are, by chance, unlikely to always get perfect agreement to the ratio in the population. For example, even when the ratio in the population is 75:25, some samples will have that ratio, but you are also likely to get 76:24, 74:26, 77:23, 73:27 etc. The range of possible outcomes among 100 offspring goes all the way from 0:100 to 100:0. So the distribution of the chi-square statistic generated by taking samples in two categories from a population in which there really is a ratio of 75:25 will look like the one in Figure 5.2, and the most unlikely 5% of outcomes will generate values of the statistic

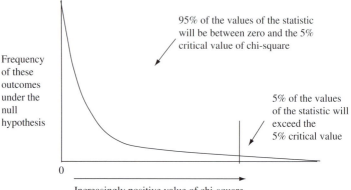

Figure 5.2   The distribution of the chi-square statistic generated by taking samples from a population containing only two categories in a known ratio. Most of the samples will have the same ratio as the expected and thus generate a chi-square statistic of zero, but the remainder will differ from this by chance, thus giving positive values of chi-square. The most extreme 5% departures from the expected ratio will generate statistics greater than the critical value of chi-square.

that will be greater than a critical value determined by the number of independent categories in the analysis.

Going back to the result of the genetic experiment given above, the expected numbers are 75 and 25 and the observed numbers are 86 brown and 14 albino.

To get the value of chi-square, you calculate:

$$\chi^2 = \frac{(86 - 75)^2}{75} + \frac{(14 - 25)^2}{25} = 6.453$$

The critical 5% value of chi-square for an analysis of two independent categories is 3.841. This means that only the most extreme 5% of departures from the expected ratio will generate a chi-square statistic **greater than this value** (I have not given a table of critical values of chi-square, because statistical packages now give both the statistic and its probability). There will be more about the chi-square test in Chapter 17.

Since the actual value of chi-square is 6.453, the observed result is significantly different to the result expected under the null hypothesis. The researcher would conclude that the ratio in the population sampled is not 3:1 and therefore reject the null hypothesis.

5.9 What if you get a statistic with a probability of exactly 0.05?

Many statistics texts do not mention this and students often ask, 'What if you get a probability of **exactly 0.05**?' Here the result would be considered **not significant**, since significance has been defined as a probability of **less than 0.05** (<0.05). Some texts define a significant result as one where the probability is **less than or equal to 0.05** (≤0.05). In practice this will make very little difference, but since Fisher proposed the 'less than 0.05' definition, which is also used by most scientific publications, it will be used here.

More importantly, many researchers would be uneasy about any result with a probability close to 0.05 and would be likely to repeat the experiment because it is so close to the critical value. If the null hypothesis applies, then there is a 0.95 probability of a non-significant result on any trial, so you would be unlikely to get a similarly marginal result when you repeated the experiment.

5.10 Statistical significance and biological significance

It is important to realise that a statistically significant result may not necessarily have any biological significance. Here is an example. A large study of male college students aged 21 was used to compare the sperm counts of 5000 coffee drinkers with 5000 non-coffee drinkers. Results showed that the coffee drinkers had fewer viable sperm per millilitre of semen than non-coffee drinkers and this difference was significant at $P < 0.05$. Nevertheless, a follow-up study of the same males over the next 15 years showed no difference in their effective fertility, as measured by the number of children produced by the partners of each group. Therefore, at least in terms of fertility, the difference was not biologically significant.

If you get a significant result you need to ask yourself, 'What does this mean biologically?' This is another aspect of realism, which was first discussed in relation to experimental design in Chapter 4.

5.11 Summary and conclusion

All statistical tests are a way of obtaining the probability of a particular outcome. This probability is either generated directly as shown in the 'beads from a sack' example, or a test that generates a statistic (e.g. the chi-square test) is applied to the data. A test statistic is just a number that usually increases as the difference between an observed and expected value (or between samples) also increases. As the value of the statistic becomes larger and larger, the probability of an event generating that statistic gets smaller and smaller. Once the probability of that event or one more extreme is less than 5%, it is concluded that the outcome is statistically significant.

A range of tests will be covered in the rest of this book, but all of them are really just methods for obtaining the probability of an outcome that helps you make a decision about your hypothesis. Nevertheless, it is important to realise that the probability of the result does not make a decision for you, and that even a statistically significant result may not necessarily have any biological significance – the result has to be considered in relation to the system you are investigating.

6 | Working from samples – data, populations, and statistics

6.1 Using a sample to infer the characteristics of a population

Usually you cannot study the whole population, so every time you gather data from a sample you are 'working in the dark' because the sample may not be very representative of that population. You have to take every possible precaution, including having a good sampling design, to try to ensure a representative sample. Unfortunately you still do not know whether it **is** representative! Although it is dangerous to extrapolate to the more general case from measurements on a subset of individuals, that is what researchers have to do whenever they cannot work on the entire population.

This chapter discusses statistical methods for estimating the characteristics of a population from a sample, and explains how these estimates can be used for significance testing.

6.2 Statistical tests

Statistical tests can be divided into two groups, called **parametric** and **non-parametric** tests. Parametric tests make certain assumptions, including that the data fit a known distribution. In most cases this is a **normal distribution** (see below). These tests are used for ratio, interval, or ordinal scale variables. Non-parametric tests do not make so many assumptions. There is a wide range of non-parametric tests available for ratio, interval, ordinal, or nominal scale variables.

6.3 The normal distribution

A lot of variables, especially 'biological' ones, tend to be normally distributed. For example, if you measure the height of the entire adult female population of a large city and plot the frequency of individuals against their height, the distribution will look like a symmetrical bell, which has been called the **normal distribution** (Figure 6.1).

The normal distribution has been found to apply to many physiological variables (e.g. the number of erythrocytes per millilitre of blood, resting heart rate, reaction time and skull diameter). It also applies to an enormous number of other variables in nature (e.g. the maximum speed at which people can run, the initial growth rate of colonies of the mould *Aspergillus niger* on laboratory agar plates, the shell length of many species of marine snails, the number of abalone per square kilometre of seagrass, or the number of sap-sucking bugs per tomato plant).

The very useful thing about normally distributed variables is that two **descriptive statistics** – the **mean** and the **standard deviation** – can describe this distribution. From these, you can predict the proportion of data that will be less than or greater than a particular value. Consequently, tests that use the properties of the normal distribution are straightforward, powerful, and easy to apply. To use them you have to be sure your data are reasonably 'normal'. (There are methods to assess normality and these will be described later.)

To understand parametric tests you need to be familiar with some statistics used to describe the normal distribution and some of its properties.

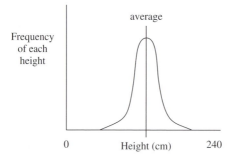

Figure 6.1 An example of a normally distributed population. The shape of the distribution is symmetrical about the average and the majority of values are close to the average, with an upper and lower 'tail' of relatively tall and relatively short people respectively.

6.3.1   The mean of a normally distributed population

First, the mean (the average) symbolised by the Greek μ describes the location of the centre of the normal distribution. It is the sum of all the values (X_1, X_2 etc.) divided by the population size (N). The formula for the mean is:

$$\mu = \frac{\sum\limits_{i=1}^{N} X_i}{N} \tag{6.1}$$

This formula needs some explanation. It contains some common standard abbreviations and symbols. First, the symbol Σ means 'the sum of'.

The symbol X_i means, 'All the X values specified by the restrictions listed below and above the Σ symbol.' The lowest value of i is specified underneath Σ (here it is 1, meaning the first value in the data set for the population) and the highest is specified above Σ (here it is N, which is the last value in the data set for the population). The horizontal line means that the quantity above this line is divided by the quantity below. Therefore, you add up all the values (X_1 to X_N) and then divide this number by the size of the population (N).

(Some textbooks use Y instead of X. From Chapter 3 you will recall that some data can be expressed as two-dimensional graphs with an X and Y axis. Here I will use X and show distributions with a mean on the X axis, but later in this book you will meet cases of data that can be thought of as values of Y with distributions on the Y axis.)

As a quick example of the calculation of a mean, here is a population of only four snails ($N = 4$). The shell lengths in mm of these four individuals (X_1 through to X_4) are 6, 7, 9, and 10, so the mean, μ, is $32 \div 4 = 8$ mm.

6.3.2   The variance of a population

The mean describes the location of the centre of the normal distribution, but two populations can have the same mean but very different dispersions around their means. For example, a population of four snails with shell lengths of 1, 2, 9, and 10 mm will have the same mean, but greater dispersion, than another population with shell lengths of 5, 5, 6, and 6 mm.

There are several ways of indicating dispersion. The **range**, which is just the difference between the lowest and highest value in the population, is sometimes used. However, the **variance**, symbolised by the Greek σ^2, provides a lot of information about the normal distribution that can be used in statistical tests.

To calculate the variance you first calculate μ. Then, by subtraction, you calculate the difference between each value $(X_1, \ldots, X_N)$ and μ, square these differences (to convert each to a positive quantity) and add them together to get the sum of the squares, which is then divided by the sample size. This is similar to the way the average is calculated, but here you have **an average value for the dispersion.**

This procedure is shown pictorially in Figure 6.2 for the population of only four snails, with shell lengths of 6, 7, 9, and 10 cm, followed by the formula for the variance.

The formula for the above procedure is straightforward:

$$\sigma^2 = \frac{\sum\limits_{i=1}^{N} (X_i - \mu)^2}{N} \tag{6.2}$$

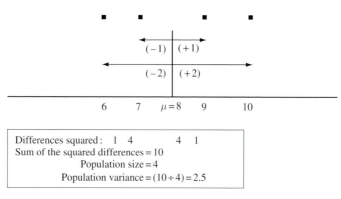

Differences squared: 1 4   4 1
Sum of the squared differences = 10
Population size = 4
Population variance = (10 ÷ 4) = 2.5

Figure 6.2 Calculation of the variance of a population consisting of only four individuals with shell lengths of 6, 7, 9, and 10 mm, each indicated by the symbol ■. The vertical line shows the mean μ. Horizontal arrows show the difference between each value and the mean. The numbers in brackets are the magnitude of each difference, and the contents of the box show these differences squared, their sum, and the variance obtained by dividing the sum of the squared differences by the population size.

If there is no dispersion at all, the variance will be zero (every X value will be the same and equal to μ, so the top line in the equation above will be zero). The variance will increase as the dispersion of the values about the mean increases.

6.3.3   The standard deviation of a population

The importance of the variance is apparent when you obtain the standard deviation, which is symbolised for a population by σ and is just the square root of the variance. For example, if the variance is 64, the standard deviation is 8.

The standard deviation is important because the mean of a normally distributed population, plus or minus one standard deviation, includes 68.27% of the values within that population.

Even more importantly, 95% of the values in the population will be within ± 1.96 standard deviations of the mean. This is especially important since the remaining 5% of values will be outside this range and therefore further away from the mean (Figure 6.3). Remember from Chapter 5 that 5% is the commonly used significance level.

These two statistics are all you need to describe the location and shape of a normal distribution and can also be used to determine the proportion of the population that is less than or more than a particular value. There is an example in Box 6.1.

6.3.4   The Z statistic

The proportions of the normal distribution described in the previous section can be expressed in a different and more workable way. For a normal distribution the difference between any value and the mean,

---

Box 6.1 Use of the standard normal distribution

For a normally distributed population with a mean height of 170 cm and a standard deviation of 10, 95% of the individuals in that population will have heights within the range of $170 \pm (1.96 \times 10)$ (which is 150.4 to 189.6 cm). You only have a 5% chance of finding someone who is either taller than 189.6 cm or shorter than 150.4 cm.

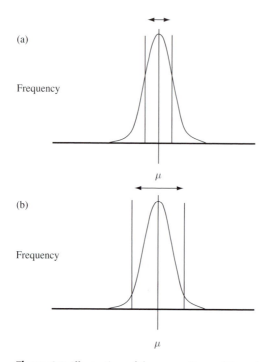

Figure 6.3 Illustration of the proportions of the values in a normally distributed population. (a) 68.27% of values are within ± 1 standard deviation from the mean and (b) 95% of values are within ± 1.96 standard deviations from the mean. These percentages correspond to the area of the distribution enclosed by the two vertical lines.

divided by the standard deviation, gives a ratio called the **Z statistic** that is also normally distributed, with a mean of zero and a standard deviation of 1.00. This is called the **standard normal distribution**:

$$Z = \frac{X_i - \mu}{\sigma} \qquad (6.3)$$

Consequently, the value of the Z statistic specifies the number of standard deviations it is from the mean. In the case of the example in Box 6.1 above, a value of 189.6 cm is $\dfrac{189.6 - 170}{10} = 1.96$ standard deviations away from the mean.

In contrast, a value of 175 cm is $\dfrac{175 - 170}{10} = 0.5$ standard deviations away from the mean.

Once this ratio is greater than $+1.96$ or less than -1.96 the probability of obtaining that value of X is less than 5%. The Z statistic will be discussed again later in this chapter.

6.4 Samples and populations

The equations for the mean, variance, and standard deviation given above apply to a **population** – the case where you have obtained data for every individual present. For a population the values of μ, σ^2, and σ are called **parameters** or **population statistics** and are true values (assuming no mistakes in measurement or calculation).

When you take a **sample** from a population and calculate the sample mean, sample variance and sample standard deviation, these are **true values for that sample** but are only **estimates** of μ, σ^2, and σ. Consequently, they are given different symbols (the Roman $\bar{X}$, s^2, and s respectively) and are called **sample statistics**. But remember – since these statistics are only estimates they may not be accurate measures of the true population statistics.

6.4.1 The sample mean

First, the procedure for calculating a sample mean is the same as for calculating the population mean, except (as mentioned above) the sample mean is symbolised by $\bar{X}$ because it is only an estimate of μ.

The sample mean is:

$$\bar{X} = \frac{\sum_{i=1}^{n} X_i}{n} \qquad (6.4)$$

(Note that the lower case n is used to indicate the sample size, compared with the capital N used to indicate the population size in equation (6.1.))

6.4.2 The sample variance

When you calculate the sample variance this estimate of σ^2 is also likely to be subject to error. Small sample size also introduces a consistent bias, but this can be compensated for by a modification to equation (6.2). For a population the variance is:

$$\sigma^2 = \frac{\sum\limits_{i=1}^{N} (X_i - \mu)^2}{N}$$ (6.5) copied from (6.2)

In contrast, the sample variance is estimated using the following formula:

$$s^2 = \frac{\sum\limits_{i=1}^{n} (X_i - \bar{X})^2}{n-1}$$ (6.6)

Note that the sum of squares is divided by $n-1$, when you would expect it to be divided by n. This is to reduce a bias caused by small sample size, and which is easily explained by an example. Imagine you wanted to estimate the population variance of the height of all adult females in a population of 10 000 by sampling only 100. This small sample is unlikely to include a sufficient proportion of people who are in either the upper or lower extremes of height within that population (the really short and really tall people), because there are relatively few of them. They will, nevertheless, make a big contribution to the population variance because they are so far from the mean (the value of $(X_i - \mu)^2$ will be a large quantity for every one of those individuals). So the sample variance will tend to underestimate the population variance and needs to be corrected.

To illustrate this I ask my students to look around the lecture room and ask themselves, 'Are there any extremely tall or very short people present?' (The answer so far has been, 'No.' One day, depending on who shows up to my classes, I may have to choose a different variable). To make s^2 the best possible estimate of σ^2, you need to divide the sum of squares by $n-1$, not n. This correction will make the sample variance (and sample standard deviation) larger.

Note that this correction will have a considerable effect when n is small (imagine dividing by 3 instead of 4) but less effect as sample size increases (imagine dividing by 999 instead of 1000). Less correction is needed as sample size increases because larger samples are more likely to include individuals from the extremes of the population you are sampling.

Here you may be thinking, 'Why don't I have to correct the mean in this way as well?' You do not have to because you are equally likely to miss out on sampling both the positive and negative extremes in the population.

6.5   Your sample mean may not be an accurate estimate of the population mean

A sample mean ($\bar{X}$) may, or may not, be an accurate estimation of the true population mean μ. Estimates from small samples are especially likely to be inaccurate, simply by chance.

To illustrate this, if you take a lot of samples of a certain size (n) at random from a population and calculate the **mean** of each sample, they are unlikely to all be the same. Instead the sample means will be dispersed around the population mean μ.

Statisticians have shown that the distribution of these sample means is also normal **with its own mean (which is also μ), variance**, and **standard deviation.**

The standard deviation of the distribution of sample means is an extremely important statistic. It is called **the standard error of the mean** (or the **standard error**, or abbreviated as **SEM** or **SE**) and given the symbol $\sigma_{\bar{X}}$ to distinguish it from the sample standard deviation (s) and the population standard deviation (σ). Importantly, **as sample size increases the standard error of the mean decreases** and therefore the accuracy of any single estimate of the population mean is likely to improve. This is shown in Figure 6.4.

It is useful to know how precise your estimate ($\bar{X}$) of μ is likely to be for a certain sample size. When you take a lot of samples, each of size n, from a population whose parametric statistics are known (as illustrated in Figure 6.4) the **standard error of the mean** can be estimated by dividing the standard deviation of the population by the square root of the sample size (n):

$$\text{SEM} = \sigma_{\bar{X}} = \frac{\sigma}{\sqrt{n}} \tag{6.7}$$

A numerical example is given in Table 6.1, which clearly illustrates that the means of larger samples are likely to be relatively close to the population mean.

The standard error of the mean is important because it can be used to calculate the range within which a particular percentage of the sample means will occur. Since the sample means are normally distributed with a mean of μ, then $\mu \pm 1$ SEM will include 68.27% of the sample means and $\mu \pm 1.96$ SEM will include 95% of the sample means.

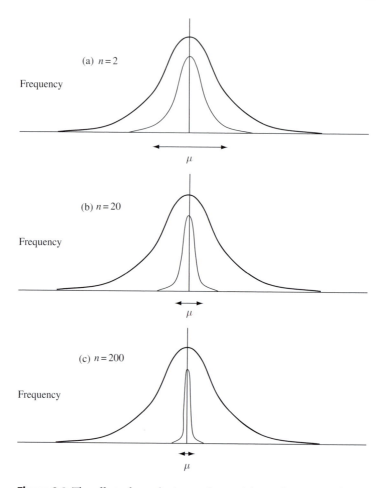

Figure 6.4 The effect of sample size on the precision and accuracy of values of $\bar{X}$ as estimates of μ. The heavy line shows the distribution of a population with parametric mean μ. The lighter line shows the distribution of the means of 200 independent samples, each of which has a sample size of (a) 2, (b) 20, and (c) 200. Note that the distribution of the means is normal with a mean of μ and that the expected range of the sample means decreases as sample size increases. The double-headed arrow shows the range within which 95% of the sample means are expected to occur.

Table 6.1. A numerical example of the effect of sample size on the accuracy and precision of values of $\bar{X}$ obtained by taking random samples of size 2, 20, or 200 from a population with a known variance of 600. As sample size increases the values of the sample means become much closer to the population mean. Precision improves and therefore the sample means will tend to be more accurate estimates of μ

Population parameters				
Variance σ^2	σ	Sample size (n)	$\sqrt{n}$	Standard error of the mean $\left(\frac{\sigma}{\sqrt{n}}\right)$
600	24.49	2	1.41	17.32
600	24.49	20	4.47	5.48
600	24.49	200	14.14	1.73

This can also be expressed as a ratio. The difference between any sample mean $\bar{X}$ and the population mean μ, divided by the standard error of the mean:

$$\frac{\bar{X} - \mu}{\sigma_{\bar{X}}} \tag{6.8}$$

will give the Z statistic already discussed in Section 6.3.4, with a mean of zero and a standard deviation of 1.00. As the difference between $\bar{X}$ and μ increases the value of Z will become increasingly positive (if $\bar{X}$ is greater than μ) or increasingly negative (if $\bar{X}$ is less than μ). Once Z is less than -1.96, or greater than $+1.96$, the probability of getting that difference between the sample mean and the known population mean μ is less than 5% (Figure 6.5).

This formula can be used to test hypotheses about the means of samples when population parameters are known. Box 6.2 gives a worked example.

6.6   What do you do when you only have data from one sample?

As shown above, the standard error of the mean is very important for hypothesis testing because it can be used to predict the range around μ within which 95% of means of a certain sample size will occur.

Unfortunately, a researcher usually does not know the true values of the population parameters μ and σ **because they only have a sample,** and statistical decisions have to be made from the limited information provided

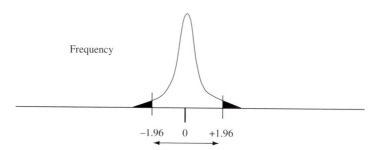

Figure 6.5 Distribution of the Z statistic (the ratio of $\frac{\bar{X} - \mu}{\text{SEM}}$ obtained by taking the means of a large number of small samples from a normal distribution). By chance 95% of the sample means will be within the range -1.96 to $+1.96$ (the unshaded area), with the remaining 5% outside this range (the two symmetrical shaded areas).

by that sample. Here too, knowing the standard error of the mean would be extremely helpful!

If you only have data from a sample, you can calculate the sample mean ($\bar{X}$), the sample variance (s^2) and sample standard deviation (s). These are your **best estimates** of the population statistics μ, σ, and σ^2. Therefore you can use s to estimate the standard error of the mean by substituting s for σ in equation (6.7). This is also called the standard error of the mean and abbreviated as 'SEM':

Box 6.2 Use of the Z statistic

The known population value of μ is 100 and σ is 36. You take a sample of 16 individuals and obtain a sample mean of 81. What is the probability that this sample mean is the same as the population mean?

$\mu = 100$, $\sigma = 36$, $n = 16$, so the $\sqrt{n} = 4$, and the $\text{SEM} = \frac{\sigma}{\sqrt{n}} = \frac{36}{4} = 9$

Therefore the value of:

$$\frac{\bar{X} - \mu}{\text{SEM}} \quad \text{is} \quad \frac{81 - 100}{9} = -2 \cdot 11$$

The ratio is outside the range of ± 1.96 so the probability that the sample mean has come from a population with a mean of μ is less than 0.05. Thus, the sample mean is significantly different to the population mean.

$$s_{\bar{X}} = \frac{s}{\sqrt{n}} \tag{6.9}$$

where s is the sample standard deviation and n is the sample size. Note from equation (6.9) that the sample SEM estimated in this way has a different symbol to the SEM estimated from the population statistics ($s_{\bar{X}}$ instead of $\sigma_{\bar{X}}$).

What does this give you? The estimate of the standard error of the mean, made from your sample, can be used to predict the range around any hypothetical value of μ within which 95% of the means of all samples of size n taken from that population will occur. This is illustrated in Figure 6.6.

Therefore, in terms of making a decision about whether your sample mean differs significantly from an expected value of μ, the formula:

$$\frac{\bar{X} - \mu_{\text{expected}}}{\text{SEM}} \tag{6.10}$$

corresponds to equation (6.8), but with $s_{\bar{X}}$ used instead of $\sigma_{\bar{X}}$ as the SEM. Here it seems logical that once this ratio is <-1.96 or $>+1.96$, the difference between the sample mean and the expected value would be considered statistically significant at the 5% level.

This is an appropriate procedure, **but a correction is needed**, especially for samples of less than 100, which are very prone to sampling error and therefore likely to give poor estimates of the population mean, standard

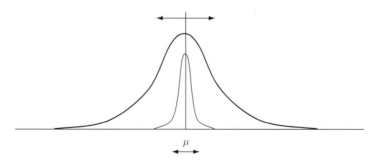

Figure 6.6 If you only have one sample, you can calculate the standard deviation, s, which is your only estimate of the population standard deviation σ. You can estimate the standard error of the mean of the population by dividing the sample standard deviation by the square root of the sample size (equation (6.9)). The lower shorter double-headed arrow shows the range within which 95% of the means of all samples of size n taken from a population with an hypothetical mean of μ would be expected to occur.

deviation, and standard error of the mean. For small samples the distribution of this ratio is **wider and flatter** than the distribution obtained by
calculating the standard error of the mean from the (known) population
standard deviation. As sample size increases the distribution gets closer and
closer to the one shown in Figure 6.5 (see Figure 6.7). Therefore equation
(6.10) is appropriate, but for small samples the range within which 95% of
the values of all means will occur is wider (e.g. for a sample size of 4 the
adjusted range within which 95% of values would be expected is from
-3.182 to $+3.182$). **Using this correction, you can test hypotheses about
your sample mean $\bar{X}$ without knowing the population statistics.**

The shape of this wider and flatter distribution of the expected ratio for
small samples was established by W.S. Gossett who published his work

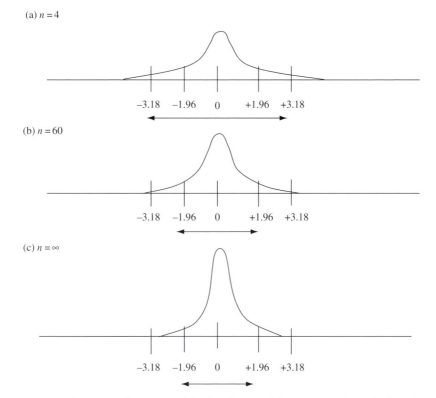

(a) $n = 4$

−3.18   −1.96   0   +1.96   +3.18

(b) $n = 60$

−3.18   −1.96   0   +1.96   +3.18

(c) $n = \infty$

−3.18   −1.96   0   +1.96   +3.18

Figure 6.7 Illustration of the distribution of the t statistic obtained when the
sample statistic s is used as an estimate of σ (a) for $n = 4$, (b) for $n = 60$, and
(c) $n = \infty$.

Table 6.2. The range of the 95% confidence interval for the t statistic in relation to sample size. (a) $n=4$, (b) $n=60$, (c) $n=200$, (d) $n=1000$, and (e) $n=\infty$. Note that the 95% confidence interval decreases as the sample size increases and that the value of t for a sample of infinite size is the same as the Z statistic. Values of t were calculated using the equations given by Zelen and Severo (1964)

	Formula	Statistic	Sample size	95% confidence interval
(a)	$\frac{\bar{X}-\mu}{s_{\bar{X}}}$	t	4	± 3.182
(b)	$\frac{\bar{X}-\mu}{s_{\bar{X}}}$	t	60	± 2.001
(c)	$\frac{\bar{X}-\mu}{s_{\bar{X}}}$	t	200	± 1.972
(d)	$\frac{\bar{X}-\mu}{s_{\bar{X}}}$	t	1000	± 1.962
(e)	$\frac{\bar{X}-\mu}{s_{\bar{X}}}$	t	∞	± 1.96

under the pseudonym of 'Student' (see Student, 1908). Consequently the distribution is often called the 'Student' distribution or 'Student's t' distribution. Two examples of the distribution of t are shown in Figure 6.7 and Table 6.2. As sample size increases the t statistic for an α of 0.05 decreases and becomes closer and closer to 1.96, which is the value for a sample of infinite size and also for the Z statistic.

6.7 Why are the statistics that describe the normal distribution so important?

Sample statistics like the mean, variance, standard deviation, and **especially** the standard error of the mean are estimates of population statistics that can be used to predict the range within which 95% of the means of a particular sample size will occur. Knowing this, you can use a parametric test to estimate the probability that a sample mean is the same as an expected value, or the probability that the means of two samples are from the same population. These tests will be described in Chapter 7.

Here you might be thinking, 'These statistical methods have the potential to be very prone to error! My sample mean may be an inaccurate estimate of μ and then I am using the sample standard deviation (s) to infer the standard error of the mean.' This is true and unavoidable when you extrapolate from only one sample, but the corrections described in this chapter and knowledge of how the sample mean is likely to become a more accurate estimate of μ as sample size increases, helps ensure that the best possible estimates are obtained.

6.8   Distributions that are not normal

Some variables do not have a normal distribution. Nevertheless, statisticians have shown that **even when a population does not have a normal distribution**, if you take repeated samples of size 25 or more, **the distribution of the means of these samples will have an approximately normal distribution with a mean μ and standard error of the mean** $\dfrac{\sigma}{\sqrt{n}}$ (which can be estimated by $\dfrac{s}{\sqrt{n}}$), just as they do when the population is normal (Figure 6.8). Furthermore,

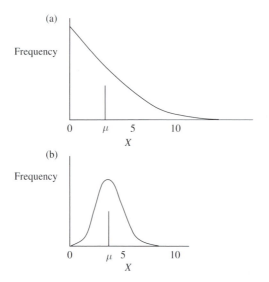

Figure 6.8 An example of the central limit theorem. Even if a population does not have a normal distribution, the means of samples of size 25 (or greater) from that population will have an approximately normal distribution with mean μ and standard error of $\dfrac{\sigma}{\sqrt{n}}$ (which can be estimated from a sample by $\dfrac{s}{\sqrt{n}}$). (a) Distribution of a population that is not normal, with mean μ and standard deviation σ. (b) The distribution of the means of 200 samples, each of $n = 25$ taken at random from the population shown in (a), is approximately normal with a mean of μ and standard error of $\dfrac{\sigma}{\sqrt{n}}$.

for populations that are approximately normal, this even holds for sample sizes as small as five. This property, which is called the **central limit theorem**, makes it possible to use some parametric tests on data from non-normal populations, provided you have a reasonably sized sample.

For data that are grossly non-normal, and for nominal scale data, **non-parametric** tests have been developed. These can be used with a wide range of data, including normally distributed data, and will be discussed later in this book. You have already met a non-parametric test for categorical data in Chapter 5 when the chi-square test was used to compare the observed and expected proportions in two categories.

6.9   Other distributions

Not all data are normally distributed. Sometimes a frequency distribution may resemble a normal distribution and be symmetrical, but is much flatter (Figure 6.9(b)). This type of distribution is **platykurtic**. In contrast, a distribution that resembles a normal distribution but has too many values around the mean and in the tails is **leptokurtic** (Figure 6.9(c)).

If the distribution is similar to a normal one but not symmetrical in that one of the tails of the distribution extends further than the other, it is **skewed**. If the upper tail is longer the distribution has a **positive skew** (Figure 6.9(d))

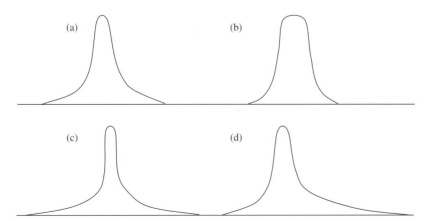

Figure 6.9 Distributions that are similar to the normal distribution. (a) A normal distribution, (b) a platykurtic distribution, (c) a leptokurtic distribution, (d) positive skew.

and if the lower tail is longer, it has a **negative skew**. Other distributions include the binomial distribution and the Poisson distribution.

The binomial distribution has already been mentioned in Chapter 5. If a population can be partitioned into two categories (e.g. black and white beads in a sack), then the probability of sampling **either** category is 1.0 and the probability of sampling a particular category will be its proportion in the population (e.g. 0.5 for a population where half the beads are black and half are white). The proportions of each of the two categories in samples containing two or more individuals will follow a pattern called the binomial distribution. Table 5.2 gave the expected distribution of the proportions of two colours in samples where $n = 6$ from a population containing 50% black and 50% white beads.

The Poisson distribution applies when you sample something by examining randomly chosen patches of a certain size, within which there is a very low probability of finding what you are looking for, so most of your data will have the value of zero. Here is an example. Koala bears are not common in most parts of Queensland and you can walk through some areas of forest for days without seeing one. If you sample a large number of randomly chosen patches, each one square kilometre in area, you will generally record no koalas. Sometimes, however, you will find one koala, even more rarely two, and, very rarely indeed, three or more. This will generate a Poisson distribution where most values are zero, a few are '1' and even fewer are '2' and '3' etc.

6.10   Other statistics that describe a distribution

Although the mean and standard deviation are the most commonly used descriptive statistics, there are others that describe a distribution.

6.10.1 The median

The median is the middle value of a set of data listed in order of magnitude. For example, a sample with the values 1, 6, 3, 9, 4, 11, and 16 is ranked in order as 1, 3, 4, 6, 9, 11, and 16, and the middle value is 6. You can calculate the location of the value of the median using the formula:

$$M = X_{(n+1)/2} \tag{6.11}$$

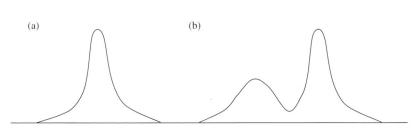

Figure 6.10 (a) A unimodal distribution. (b) A bimodal distribution.

Which means, 'The median is the value of X whose numbered position in an ordered sequence corresponds to the sample size plus one, and then divided by two.' For the sample of seven listed above the median is the fourth value, X_4, which is 6. For even-sized samples the median will lie between two values (e.g. $X_{5.5}$) in which case it is the average of the value below (X_5) and above it (X_6). The procedure becomes more complex when there are tied values, but most statistical packages will calculate the median of a set of data.

6.10.2 The mode

The mode is defined as the most frequently occurring value in a set of data, so a normal distribution has only one mode. Sometimes, however, a distribution may have two or more clearly separated peaks in which case it is bimodal or multimodal respectively (Figure 6.10).

6.10.3 The range

The range is the difference between the largest and smallest value in a sample or population. The range of the set of data in Section 6.10.1 is $16 - 1 = 15$.

6.11   Conclusion

The mean and the standard deviation are sufficient to describe the shape of a normal distribution. The sample statistics $\bar{X}$ and s provide estimates of the population statistics μ and σ. Importantly, the distribution of the means of samples from a normal population is also normal, with a mean of μ and a standard error of $\dfrac{\sigma}{\sqrt{n}}$ that can be estimated from a sample of two or more by $\dfrac{s}{\sqrt{n}}$. This allows you to use the properties of the normal distribution to predict the range around $\bar{X}$ (your best and only estimate of μ) within which 95% (or 99% or 99.9% if required) of the means of all samples of size n taken from that population will occur.

Even more importantly, when the population of the variable you have measured is not normally distributed, the distribution of the means of samples of about 25 or more will be approximately normal, with a mean of μ and a standard error of $\dfrac{\sigma}{\sqrt{n}}$. This also provides a way of predicting the range of values within which there is a 95% probability that any sample mean of size n will occur. In the next chapter some very straightforward tests that use this property of the normal distribution of sample means will be described.

7 | Normal distributions – tests for comparing the means of one and two samples

7.1 Introduction

Sample statistics such as $\bar{X}$ and s are only estimates of population statistics but it is still possible to use these to make statistical decisions. First, as sample size increases, sample statistics are likely to become increasingly accurate estimates of population statistics. Second, as described in Chapter 6, the distribution of the means of samples of a particular size (n) taken from a normal population with population statistics of μ and σ will also be normal, with a mean of μ and a standard error of the mean of $\frac{\sigma}{\sqrt{n}}$ that can be estimated from a sample by $\frac{s}{\sqrt{n}}$. Even more usefully, provided you have a sample size of about 25 or more, these properties of the distribution of sample means apply even when the population they have been taken from is not normal, provided it is not grossly non-normal (e.g. a distribution which is bimodal). Therefore, you can often use a parametric test to make decisions about sample means even when the population you have sampled is not normally distributed.

In this chapter these concepts are used to describe how some parametric tests for comparing the means of one and two samples actually work. The first test is for comparing a single sample mean to a known population mean. The second is for comparing a single sample mean to an hypothesised value. These are followed by tests for comparing the means of two samples.

7.2 The 95% confidence interval and 95% confidence limits

In Chapter 6 it was discussed how 95% of the means of samples size n, taken from a population with a known μ and σ, would be expected to occur **within** the range of $\mu \pm 1.96 \times \text{SEM}$. This range is called the **95% confidence interval**, and the actual numbers that show the limits of that range ($\mu \pm 1.96 \times \text{SEM}$) are called the **95% confidence limits.**

If you only have data for one sample of size n, then the sample standard deviation s is your best estimate of σ and it can be used with the appropriate t statistic to calculate the 95% confidence interval for an expected or hypothesised value of μ. You have to use the formula $\mu_{\text{expected}} \pm t \times \text{SEM}$ because the population statistics are not known. This formula will give a wider confidence interval than if population statistics are known because the value of t for a finite sample size is always greater than 1.96, especially for small samples (Chapter 6).

7.3   Using the Z statistic to compare a sample mean and population mean when population statistics are known

This test uses the Z statistic to give the probability that a sample mean has been taken from a population with a known mean and standard deviation. From the population statistics μ and σ you can calculate the expected standard error of the mean $\left(\frac{\sigma}{\sqrt{n}}\right)$ for a sample of size of n and therefore the 95% confidence interval (Figure 7.1), which is the range within $\mu \pm 1.96 \times \text{SEM}$. If your sample mean, $\bar{X}$, occurs within this range, the probability it has come from the population with mean μ is 0.05 or greater, **so the mean of the population from which the sample has been taken is not significantly different to the known population mean.** If, however, your sample mean occurs outside the confidence interval, the probability it has been taken from the population of mean μ is less than 0.05, **so the mean of the population from which the sample has been taken is significantly different to the known population mean μ.**

This is a very straightforward test (Figure 7.1). If you decide on a probability level other than 0.05, you simply need to use a different value than 1.96 (e.g. for the 99% confidence interval you would use 2.576).

Although you could calculate the 95% confidence limits every time you made this type of comparison, it is far easier to calculate the ratio $Z = \frac{\bar{X} - \mu}{\text{SEM}}$ as described in Section 6.3.4. All this formula does is divide the distance between the sample mean and the known population mean by

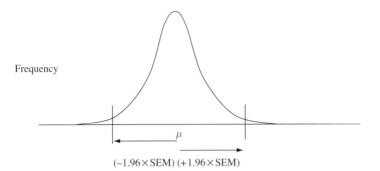

Figure 7.1 The 95% confidence interval, obtained by taking the means of a large number of small samples from a normally distributed population with known statistics, is indicated by the horizontal distance enclosed within $\mu \pm 1.96$ SEM. The remaining 5% of sample means are expected to be further away from μ. Therefore, a sample mean that lies **inside** the confidence interval will be considered to have come from the population with a mean of μ, while a sample mean that lies **outside** the 95% confidence interval will be considered to have come from a population with a mean significantly different to μ, assuming an α of 0.05.

the standard error, so, once the value of Z is <-1.96 or $>+1.96$, the mean of the population from which the sample has been taken is considered significantly different to the known population mean, assuming an α of 0.05.

Here you may be wondering if a population mean could ever be known, apart from small populations where every individual has been censused. Sometimes, however, researchers have so many data for a particular variable that they consider the sample statistics indicate the true values of population statistics. For example, many physiological variables such as the number of red (or white) blood cells per ml, fasting blood glucose levels, and resting body temperature have been measured on several million healthy people. This sample is so large it can be considered to give extremely accurate estimates of the population statistics. Remember, as sample size increases, $\bar{X}$ becomes closer and closer to the true population mean and the correction of $n - 1$ used to calculate the standard deviation also becomes less and less important. There is an example of the comparison between a sample mean and a 'known' population mean in Box 7.1.

Box 7.1 Comparison between a sample mean and a known population mean where population parameters are known

The mean number of white blood cells per ml of blood in healthy adults is 7500 per ml, with a standard deviation of 1250. These statistics are from a sample of over one million people and are therefore considered to be the population statistics μ and σ.

Ten astronauts who had spent six months in space had their white cell counts measured as soon as they returned to Earth. The data are shown below. What is the probability that the sample mean $\bar{X}$ has been taken from the healthy population?

The white cell counts are: 7130, 6845, 7055, 7235, 7200, 7450, 7750, 7950, 7340, and 7150 cells/ml.

The population statistics for healthy human adults are $\mu = 7500$ and $\sigma = 1250$

The sample size $n = 10$
The sample mean $\bar{X} = 7310.5$
The standard error of the mean $= \frac{\sigma}{\sqrt{n}} = \frac{1,250}{\sqrt{10}} = 395.3$

Therefore, $1.96 \times \text{SEM} = 1.96 \times 395.3 = 774.76$ and the 95% confidence interval for the means of samples of $n = 10$ is 7500 ± 774.76, which is from 6725.24 to 8274.76.

Since the mean white cell count of the ten astronauts lies within the range in which 95% of means with $n = 10$ would be expected to occur by chance, the probability that the sample mean has come from the healthy population with mean μ is not significant.

Expressed as a formula:

$$Z = \frac{\bar{X} - \mu}{\text{SEM}} = \frac{7310.5 - 7500}{395.3} = \frac{-189.5}{395.3} = -0.4794$$

Here too, since the Z value lies within the range of ± 1.96, the mean of the population from which the sample has been taken does not differ significantly from the mean of the healthy population. (The negative value is caused by the sample mean being less than the population mean.)

7.4   Comparing a sample mean with an expected value

The single sample t test compares a single sample mean to an expected value of the population mean. When population statistics are not known, the sample standard deviation s is your best and only estimate of σ for the population from which it has been taken. You can still use the 95% confidence interval of the mean, estimated from the sample standard deviation, and the t statistic described in Chapter 6 to predict the range around an expected value of μ within which 95% of the means of samples of size n taken from that population will occur. Here too, once the sample mean lies outside the 95% confidence interval, the probability of it being from a population with a mean of μ_{expected} is less than 0.05 (Figure 7.2).

Expressed as a formula, as soon as the ratio of $t = \frac{\bar{X} - \mu_{\text{expected}}}{\text{SEM}}$ is less than the critical 5% value of $-t$ or greater than $+t$, then the sample mean is considered to have come from a population with a mean significantly different to μ_{expected}.

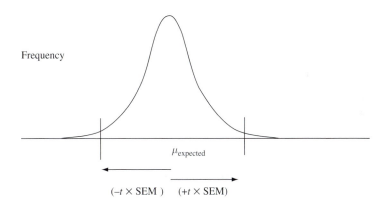

Figure 7.2 The 95% confidence interval, estimated from one sample of size n by using the t statistic, is indicated by the horizontal distance enclosed within $\mu \pm t \times \text{SEM}$. Therefore, 5% of the means of samples size n from the population would be expected to lie outside this range. If $\bar{X}$ lies inside the confidence interval, it will be considered to have come from a population with a mean the same as μ_{expected}, but if it lies outside the confidence interval, it will be considered to have come from a population with a significantly different mean, assuming an α of 0.05.

Table 7.1. Critical values of the distribution of t. The column on the far left gives the number of degrees of freedom (v). The remaining columns give the critical value of t. For example, the third column, shown in bold and headed $\alpha(2) = 0.05$, gives the 5% critical values. Note that the 5% probability value of t for a sample of infinite size (the last row) is 1.96 and thus equal to the 5% probability value for the Z distribution. Critical values were calculated using the methods given by Zelen and Severo (1964)

Degrees of freedom v	$\alpha(2) = 0.10$ or $\alpha(1) = 0.05$	$\alpha(2) = 0.05$ or $\alpha(1) = 0.025$	$\alpha(2) = 0.02$ or $\alpha(1) = 0.01$	$\alpha(2) = 0.01$ or $\alpha(1) = 0.005$
1	6.314	12.706	31.821	63.657
2	2.920	4.303	6.965	9.925
3	2.353	3.182	4.541	5.841
4	2.132	2.776	3.747	4.604
5	2.015	2.571	3.365	4.032
6	1.943	2.447	3.143	3.707
7	1.895	2.365	2.998	3.499
8	1.860	2.306	2.896	3.355
9	1.833	2.262	2.821	3.250
10	1.812	2.228	2.764	3.169
15	1.753	2.131	2.602	2.947
30	1.697	2.042	2.457	2.750
50	1.676	2.009	2.403	2.678
100	1.660	1.984	2.364	2.626
1000	1.646	1.962	2.330	2.581
∞	1.645	1.96	2.326	2.576

7.4.1 Degrees of freedom and looking up the appropriate critical value of t

The appropriate critical value of t for a sample is easily found in tables of this statistic, which are in most statistical texts. Table 7.1 gives a selection of values as an example. First, you need to look for the chosen probability level along the top line labelled as $\alpha(2)$. (There will shortly be an explanation for the column heading $\alpha(1)$.) Here I am using an α of 0.05 and the column giving these critical values is shown in bold.

The column on the left gives the number of **degrees of freedom,** which needs explanation. If you have a sample of size n and the mean of this sample is a specified value, then **all of the data within the sample except**

one are free to be any number at all, but the final one is fixed because the sum of the data in the sample divided by n must equal the mean.

Here is an example. If you have a specified sample mean of 4.25 and $n = 2$, then the first value in the sample is free to be any value at all, but the second must be one that gives a mean of 4.25, so it is a fixed number. Thus, the number of degrees of freedom for a sample of $n = 2$ are 1. For $n = 100$ and a specified mean (e.g. 4.25), 99 of the values are free to vary, but the final value is also determined by the requirement for the mean to be 4.25. Therefore the number of degrees of freedom are 99.

The number of degrees of freedom determines the critical value of the t statistic. For a single sample t test, if your sample size is n, then you need to use the t value that has $n - 1$ degrees of freedom. Therefore, for a sample size of 10, the degrees of freedom are 9 and the critical value of the t statistic for an α of 0.05 is 2.262 (Table 7.1). If your calculated value of t is less than -2.262 or more than 2.262, the expected probability of that outcome is <0.05. From now on, the appropriate t value will have a subscript to show the degrees of freedom (e.g. t_7 indicates 7 degrees of freedom).

7.4.2   One-tailed and two-tailed tests

All of the alternate hypotheses dealt with so far in this chapter do not specify anything other than, 'The mean of the population from which the sample has been drawn is different to an expected value' or 'The two samples are from populations with different means.' Therefore, these are **two-tailed hypotheses** because nothing is specified about the **direction** of the difference. The null hypothesis could be rejected by a difference in either a positive or negative direction.

Sometimes, however, you may have an alternate hypothesis that specifies a direction. For example, 'The mean of the population from which the sample has been taken is **greater** than an expected value' or 'The mean of the population from which sample A has been taken is **less** than the mean of the population from which sample B has been taken.' These are called **one-tailed hypotheses.**

If you have an alternate hypothesis that is directional, the null hypothesis will not just be one of no difference. For example, if the alternate hypothesis states that the mean of the population from which the sample has been taken will be **less** than an expected value, then the null should state, 'The

(a)

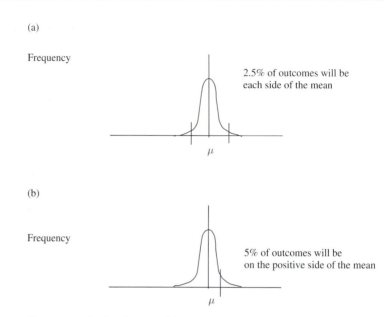

Frequency

2.5% of outcomes will be
each side of the mean

μ

(b)

Frequency

5% of outcomes will be
on the positive side of the mean

μ

Figure 7.3 The distribution of the 5% of most extreme outcomes under a two-tailed hypothesis and a one-tailed hypothesis specifying that the expected value of the mean is larger than μ. (a) The rejection regions for a two-tailed hypothesis are on both the positive and negative sides of the true population mean. (b) The rejection region for a one-tailed hypothesis occurs only on one side of the true population mean. Here it is on the right side because the hypothesis specifies that the sample mean is taken from a population with a larger mean than μ.

mean of the population from which the sample has been taken will be no different to, or **more**, than the expected value.*

You need to be cautious, however, because a directional hypothesis will affect the location of the region where the most extreme 5% of outcomes will occur. Here is an example using a single sample test where the true population mean is known. For any two-tailed hypothesis the 5% rejection region is split equally into two areas of 2.5% on the negative and positive side of μ (Figure 7.3(a)).

If, however, the hypothesis specifies that your sample is from a population with a mean that is expected to be only greater (or only less) than the true value, then in each case the most extreme 5% of possible outcomes that you would be interested in are restricted to **one side** or **one tail** of the distribution (Figure 7.3(b)).

Therefore, if you have a one-tailed hypothesis, you need to do two things to make sure you make an appropriate decision.

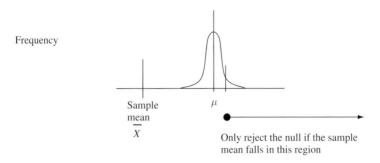

Figure 7.4 An example of the rejection region for a one-tailed test. If the alternate hypothesis states that the sample mean will be more than μ, then the null hypothesis is retained unless the sample mean lies in the region to the right, where the most extreme 5% of values would be expected to occur.

First, you need to examine your results to see if the difference is in the direction expected under the alternate hypothesis. **If it is not, then the value of the t statistic is irrelevant** – the null hypothesis will stand and the alternate hypothesis will be rejected (Figure 7.4).

Second, if the difference is in the appropriate direction, you need to choose an appropriate critical value to ensure that 5% of outcomes are concentrated in one tail of the expected distribution. This is easy. For the Z or t statistics the critical two-tailed probability of 5% is not appropriate for a one-tailed test, because it only specifies the region where 2.5% of the values will occur in each tail. So, to get the critical 5% value for a one-tailed test, you would need to use the 10% critical value for a two-tailed test. This is why the column headed $\alpha(2) = 0.10$ in Table 7.1 also includes the heading $\alpha(1) = 0.05$, and you would need to use the critical values in this column if you were doing a one-tailed test.

It is important to specify your null and alternate hypotheses, and therefore decide whether a one-or two-tailed test is appropriate, **before** you do an experiment, because the critical values are different. For example, for an α of 0.05, the two-tailed critical value for t_{10} is ± 2.228 (Table 7.1), but, if the test were one-tailed, the critical value would be **either** $+1.812$ or -1.812. So a t value of 2.0 in the correct direction would be significant for a one-tailed test but not for a two-tailed test (Figure 7.5).

Many statistical packages only give the calculated value of t (not the critical value) and its probability for a two-tailed test. In this case, however, it is even easier to obtain the one-tailed probability and you do not even

(a)

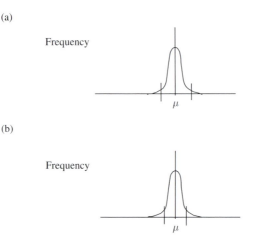

(b)

Figure 7.5 The critical value for a 5% one-tailed test is the same as the critical value for a 10% two-tailed test, except that it will be in only one tail of the distribution. (a) A two-tailed test using the 5% probability level will have a rejection region of 2.5% on both the positive and negative sides of the known population mean. The positive and negative of the critical value will define the region where the null hypothesis is rejected. (b) A one-tailed test using the 5% probability level will have a rejection region of 5% on only one side of the population mean. Therefore the 5% critical value will correspond to the value for a 10% two-tailed test, except that it will be only be either the positive or negative of the critical value, depending on the direction of the alternate hypothesis.

need a table of critical values such as Table 7.1. All you have to do is halve the two-tailed probability to get the appropriate one-tailed probability (e.g. a two-tailed probability of $P = 0.08$ is equivalent to $P = 0.04$, provided the difference is in the right direction).

If your hypothesis is one-tailed, it is appropriate to do a one-tailed test. There have, however, been cases of unscrupulous researchers who have obtained a result with a non-significant two-tailed probability (e.g. $P = 0.065$) but have then realised this would be significant if a one-tailed test were applied ($P = 0.0325$) and have subsequently modified their initial hypothesis. This is not appropriate or ethical and will be discussed in Chapter 20.

7.4.3   The application of a single sample t test

Here is an example where you might use a single sample t test. Many agricultural crops such as wheat and barley have an optimal water content for harvesting by machine. If the crop is too dry, the seed heads may shatter and be damaged, thereby reducing their value. If it is too wet, the crop may clog and damage the harvester.

The optimal desired mean water content at harvest of the rather dubious sounding crop 'Panama Gold' is 50 g/kg. Many growers sample their crop to establish whether the water content is significantly different to a desired value before making a decision to harvest.

A grower took nine 1.0 kilogram replicates at random over a widely dispersed area of their crop of Panama Gold and measured the water content of each. The data are given in Box 7.2. Is the sample likely to have come from a population where $\mu = 50\,\text{g/kg}$? The calculations are straightforward. If you analyse these data using a statistical package, the results will usually include the value of the t statistic and the probability, making it unnecessary to use a table of critical values.

Box 7.2 Comparison between a sample mean and an expected value when population statistics are not known

The water content of nine 1 kg replicates of Panama Gold taken at random from within a large field is 44, 42, 43, 49, 43, 47, 45, 46, and 43 g/kg.

The null hypothesis is that this sample is from a population with a mean water content of 50 g/kg.

The alternate hypothesis is that this sample is from a population with a mean water content that is **not** 50 g/kg.

The mean of this sample is: 44.67

The standard deviation $s = 2.29$

The standard error of the mean is $\frac{s}{\sqrt{n}} = \frac{2.29}{3} = 0.764$

Therefore $t_8 = \frac{\bar{X} - \mu_{\text{expected}}}{\text{SEM}} = \frac{44.67 - 50}{0.764} = -6.98$

Although the mean of the sample is less than the desired mean value of 50, is the difference significant? The calculated value of t_8 is -6.98. The critical value of t_8 for an α of 0.05 is ± 2.306 (Table 7.1). Therefore, the probability that the sample mean has been taken from a population with a mean water content of 50g/kg is <0.05. The grower concluded that the mean moisture content of the crop was significantly different to that of a population with a mean of 50 g/kg.

7.5   Comparing the means of two related samples

The paired sample t test is designed for cases where you have measured the same variable twice on each experimental unit under two different conditions. Some common applications of this type of comparison are measurements taken before and after drug treatments, and performance tests on athletes. Here is an example.

A sports psychologist hypothesised that athletes may perform either more or less efficiently than usual when they are first introduced to unfamiliar surroundings. They called this the 'familiarity effect'. For example, when sprinters are taken to an unfamiliar stadium it was feared they may run either faster or slower on the first day compared with the second. The familiarity effect is thought to be small, but could make the difference between achieving a world record or winning a race. There is, however, a lot of variation in running speed among individuals, so a comparison of two independent groups of different athletes might obscure any difference in speed between the first and second days. Instead, the psychologist decided to measure the running time of the **same** ten athletes over a fixed distance on the first and second day after arriving at a new stadium. The results are shown in Table 7.2.

Here the two groups are not independent because the same individuals are in each group. Nevertheless, you can generate a single independent value for each individual by taking their 'Day 1' reading away from the 'Day 2' reading. This will give a single column of differences for the ten experimental subjects, which will have its own mean and standard deviation (Table 7.2).

The null hypothesis is that there is no difference between the running times of each athlete on both days. Therefore, if the null hypothesis were true, you would expect the population of values for the **difference** for each athlete to have a mean of zero, and a standard error that can be estimated from the sample of differences by $\frac{s}{\sqrt{n}}$. **This is just another case of a single sample t test (Section** 7.4), **but here the expected population mean is zero**. Consequently, all you need to do is calculate the ratio of $\frac{\bar{X}-0}{\text{SEM}}$ and see if this statistic lies within or outside the region where 95% of the means of this sample size would be expected to occur around a population mean of zero. This has been done in Box 7.3.

Interestingly, the athletes took longer to run the same distance on the second day. Although this is a poor experimental design in that many other factors (including fatigue, differences in air temperature or wind speed)

Table 7.2. The time taken, in seconds, for ten athletes to sprint the same distance on their first and second day of running in an unfamiliar environment. The column headed 'Difference' gives the race time for Day 2 minus Day 1 for each athlete, and the sample statistics are for this column of data

Athlete number	Race time (seconds)		
	Day 1	Day 2	Difference
1	13.5	13.6	+ 0.1
2	14.6	14.6	0.0
3	12.7	12.6	− 0.1
4	15.5	15.7	+ 0.2
5	11.1	11.1	0.0
6	16.4	16.6	+ 0.2
7	13.2	13.2	0.0
8	19.3	19.5	+ 0.2
9	16.7	16.8	+ 0.1
10	18.4	18.7	+ 0.3
			$\bar{X} = 0.100$
			$s = 0.1247$
			$n = 10$
			SEM = 0.0394

Box 7.3 A worked example of a paired sample *t* test using the data from Table 7.2

$\bar{X} = 0.100$

$s = 0.12472$

$n = 10$

SEM $= 0.0394$

Therefore $t_9 = \frac{0.10 - 0}{0.03944} = 2.5355$

From Table 7.1 the critical value of t_9 is 2.262. Therefore the value of t lies outside the range within which you would expect 95% of t statistics generated by samples of $n = 9$ from a population where $\mu = 0$, so it was concluded that the mean of the population of the differences in race time was significantly different ($P < 0.05$) to an expected mean of zero.

may have confounded the results, it is consistent with the alternate hypothesis and is likely to lead to further investigation.

7.6   Comparing the means of two independent samples

Often you will need to compare the means of two independent samples. This type of comparison is particularly common when you have two randomly chosen independent samples such as a control and an experimental group, each containing different experimental units. Here the question is, 'Have the two sample means been drawn from populations with the same mean μ?'

It is easy to visualise this pictorially. Under the null hypothesis, each sample is from the same population, so 95% of the time you would expect the two sample means to lie within the 95% confidence interval surrounding μ. Here, however, you are interested in **the range of possible differences between two values of $\bar{X}$**, which will be much wider than the confidence interval for each sample, because there will be cases where one mean is at the lower end of the expected range and the other at the higher end and *vice versa* (Figure 7.6).

To obtain a *t* statistic for the difference between two independent sample means you simply need to divide $\bar{X}_A - \bar{X}_B$ by the standard error of the distribution of differences shown in Figure 7.6(b). The latter is easy to estimate because the variance of the **difference** between the means of two independent samples is the **sum** of the variances of these samples:

$$S_{A-B}^2 = S_A^2 + S_B^2 \qquad\qquad (7.1)$$

This is consistent with the much greater variance in Figure 7.6(b) compared with Figure 7.6(a). Since the SEM from a sample is $\sqrt{\frac{s^2}{n}}$, in order to get the best estimate of the standard error of $\bar{X}_A - \bar{X}_B$ you use the following formula, which is just the square root of the variance of sample A divided by the sample size of A plus the variance of sample B divided by the sample size of B:

$$\text{SEM} = \sqrt{\frac{s_A^2}{n_A} + \frac{s_B^2}{n_B}} \qquad\qquad (7.2)$$

Finally, to obtain the *t* statistic for the differences between the two means you divide $\bar{X}_A - \bar{X}_B$ by this estimate of the SEM:

(a)

Frequency

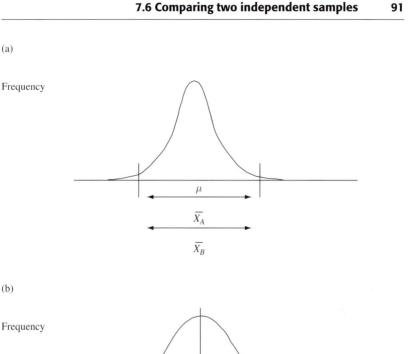

(b)

Frequency

Figure 7.6 Illustration of the comparison made by an independent sample t test. (a) The upper graph shows the range, indicated by the double-headed arrows, within which 95% of the values of means of samples size n, from a population with a mean μ, are expected to occur. (b) The lower graph shows the expected distribution of the **differences** $(\bar{X}_A - \bar{X}_B)$ between any two sample means of size n from that population. The distribution of differences will have a mean of zero (when both $\bar{X}_A$ and $\bar{X}_B$ are equal) and a much greater dispersion than in (a), because there will be cases where $\bar{X}_A$ is at the low end of the range and $\bar{X}_B$ is at the high end of the range (giving large negative values) and *vice versa* (giving large positive values). The double-headed arrow shows the 95% confidence interval for $\bar{X}_A - \bar{X}_B$. Note that it is much wider than the 95% confidence interval for the sample means shown in (a).

> **Box 7.4** A worked example of a t test for two independent samples
>
> A freshwater ecologist sampled the shell length of 15 freshwater clams in each of two lakes to see if these samples were likely to have come from populations with the same mean. The data are shown below:
>
> Lake A: 25, 40, 34, 37, 38, 35, 29, 32, 35, 44, 27, 33, 37, 38, 36
> Lake B: 45, 37, 36, 38, 49, 47, 32, 41, 38, 45, 33, 39, 46, 47, 40
> $n_A = 15$, $n_B = 15$, $\bar{X}_A = 34.67$, $\bar{X}_B = 40.87$, $s_A^2 = 24.67$, $s_B^2 = 28.69$
>
> therefore
>
> $$t_{28} = \frac{34.67 - 40.87}{\sqrt{\frac{24.67}{15} + \frac{28.69}{15}}} = \frac{-6.2}{\sqrt{1.645 + 1.913}} = -3.287$$
>
> Note that the value of t is negative, because the mean for Lake B is greater than Lake A.
>
> The critical value of t_{28} for an α of 0.05 is 2.048, so the two sample means have a less than 5% probability of being from the same population.

$$t = \frac{\bar{X}_A - \bar{X}_B}{\sqrt{\frac{s_A^2}{n_A} + \frac{s_B^2}{n_B}}} \tag{7.3}$$

Here the number of degrees of freedom is $(n_{(A)} - 1) + (n_{(B)} - 1)$, which is usually put as $(n_{(A)} + n_{(B)} - 2)$. This is because you have calculated the standard error using two independent samples, both of which have $n - 1$ degrees of freedom. You have lost a degree of freedom from each sample. A worked example is given in Box 7.4.

You may never have to manually calculate a t statistic, because statistical packages have excellent programs for doing them. But the simple worked examples in this chapter will help you understand how t tests work and will be very helpful as you continue through this book.

7.7 Are your data appropriate for a t test?

The use of a t test makes three assumptions. The first is that the data are normally distributed. The second is that each sample has been taken at random from its respective population and the third is that for an independent sample test, the variances are the same.

It has, however, been shown that *t* tests are actually very 'robust' – that is, they will still generate statistics that approximate the *t* distribution and give realistic probabilities even when the data show considerable departure from normality and when sample variances are dissimilar.

7.7.1   Assessing normality

First, if you already know that the population from which your sample has been taken is normally distributed (perhaps you have data for a variable that has been studied before), you can assume the distribution of sample means from this population will also be normally distributed.

Second, the central limit theorem discussed in Chapter 6 states that the distribution of the means of samples of about 25 or more taken from **any** population will be approximately normal, provided the population is not grossly non-normal (e.g. a population that is bimodal). Therefore, provided your sample size is sufficiently large you can usually do a parametric test.

Finally, you can examine your sample. Although there are statistical tests for normality, many statisticians (see Quinn and Keough, 2002) have cautioned that these tests often indicate the sample is significantly non-normal even when a *t* test will still give reliable results.

Some authors (e.g. Zar, 1999, Quinn and Keough, 2002) suggest plotting the cumulative frequency distribution of the sample. The easiest way to do this is to use a statistics package to give you a probability plot (often called a P-P plot). This graphs the actual cumulative frequency against the expected cumulative frequency assuming the data are normally distributed. If they are, the P-P plot will be a straight line. Any gross departures from this should be analysed cautiously and perhaps a non-parametric test used. Most statistical packages will draw a P-P plot for a sample.

7.7.2   Have the sample(s) been taken at random?

This is really just a case of having an appropriate experimental design. For a single sample test, the sample needs to have been selected at random in order to appropriately represent the population from which it has been taken. For an independent sample test, both samples need to have been selected at random.

7.7.3   Are the sample variances equal?

One easy test of whether sample variances are equal is to divide the largest by the smallest. If the samples have equal variances, this ratio will be 1.00. As the variances become more and more unequal, the value of this statistic, which is called the **F statistic** or **F ratio** after the statistician Sir Ronald A. Fisher, will increase. There will be discussion of F and tests for equality of variances in Chapters 9 and 11. Even if the variances of two samples are significantly different, you can often still apply a t test.

7.8   Distinguishing between data that should be analysed by a paired sample test or a test for two independent samples

As a researcher, or reviewer of another person's work, you may have to decide if an experimental outcome should be analysed as a paired sample test or a test for two independent samples. The way to do this is to ask, 'Are the experimental units in the two samples related or are they independent?' Here are some examples.

First, Table 7.3 shows two samples that are related – two measurements of systolic blood pressure on each member of the same group of four people given two different drugs.

Each experimental unit (person) in Table 7.3 experiences both drugs, so you would do a paired-sample test.

Table 7.3. Data for the systolic blood pressure of four people in response to Drug A and Drug B

Person	Drug A	Drug B
1	120	130
2	150	140
3	170	150
4	110	120

Table 7.4. Data for the systolic blood pressure of four people given Drug A and four people given Drug B

Person	Drug A	Drug B
1	120	
2	150	
3	160	
4	130	
5		135
6		160
7		120
8		140

An independent example is to measure blood pressure of two different groups of individuals, with each group receiving a different drug. Experimental units 1 to 4 only receive Drug A, while units 5 to 8 only receive Drug B (Table 7.4).

The samples are obviously independent. You would do an independent sample test.

7.9   Conclusion

This chapter explains how the Z test and t tests for one and two samples actually work. The concepts will help you make decisions about which test to use for a particular set of data and also be very useful when you work through the material in later chapters. They will also help you understand the results given by statistical packages.

8 | Type 1 and Type 2 errors, power, and sample size

8.1   Introduction

Every time you make a decision based on the probability of a particular result, there is a risk that your decision is wrong. There are two sorts of mistakes you can make and these are called **Type 1 error** and **Type 2 error**.

8.2   Type 1 error

A Type 1 error or **false positive** occurs when you decide the null hypothesis is false when in reality it is not. Imagine you took a sample of size n from a population with known statistics of μ and σ and subjected this sample to a particular experimental treatment. Since the population statistics are known, you could test whether this sample mean was significantly different to the population mean by doing a Z test (Section 7.3).

If the treatment had no effect, the null hypothesis would apply and your sample would simply be equivalent to one drawn at random from the population. Nevertheless, 5% of the sample means of size n will lie outside the 95% confidence interval of $\mu \pm 1.96$. Therefore, 5% of the time you would incorrectly reject the null hypothesis of no difference between your sample mean and the population mean (Figure 8.1) and accept the alternate hypothesis. This is a Type 1 error.

It is important to realise that Type 1 error can only occur when the null hypothesis applies. There is absolutely no risk if the null hypothesis is false. Unfortunately, you are most unlikely to know if the null hypothesis applies or not – if you did know, you would not be doing an experiment to test it! If the null hypothesis applies, the risk of Type 1 error is the same as the probability level you have chosen.

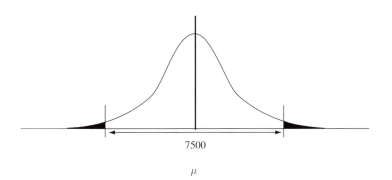

7500

μ

Figure 8.1 Illustration of Type 1 error. The known population mean is 7500 and the 95% confidence interval for the mean is shown as the double-headed horizontal arrow. There is no effect of treatment, so the distribution of sample means from the experimental population will be the same as those from the untreated population. Nevertheless, 5% of your sample means will, by chance, lie in the shaded areas outside the 95% confidence interval. Whenever a sample mean occurs in either of these areas you will incorrectly reject the null hypothesis and make a Type 1 error. This risk is unavoidable when the null hypothesis applies, but can be controlled by the chosen value of α. An α of 0.05 will have a 5% probability of Type 1 error, but an α of 0.01 will only have a 1% probability of Type 1 error.

Here, therefore, you may be thinking, 'Then why do we usually set α at 0.05? Surely an α of 0.01 or 0.001 would reduce the risk of Type 1 error?' It will, but it will affect the likelihood of Type 2 error.

8.3   Type 2 error

A Type 2 error or **false negative** occurs when you do not reject the null hypothesis, even though it is false. For the example above, this would occur when the treatment had a real effect but your experiment and analysis did not detect it.

Here is an example, using a single sample, two-tailed Z test where the population statistics are known.

8.3.1   A worked example showing Type 2 error

The population mean and variance of the number of white blood cells per millilitre in blood from healthy adults is 7500, with a standard deviation of

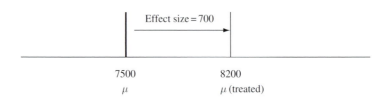

Figure 8.2 The concept of effect size displacing the population mean. The population mean, μ, is 7500 white blood cells/ml, but the drug leucoxifen increases this by 700 to 8200 cells/ml.

1250. These statistics are from more than a million people, so are considered to be the population statistics μ and σ. They were first used in Box 7.1.

Here you need to imagine the case where the new and untested experimental drug 'leucoxifen' actually causes an average increase in white blood cells of 700 per ml, so the mean of the population given leucoxifen is 700 cells/ml more than the mean of the healthy population. This change is often called the **effect size** of the treatment. Since leucoxifen is a new drug it is not known if there is an effect size or not. A researcher was asked to investigate this drug, so they administered it to a sample of several healthy people and then compared the mean white cell count of this sample with the known population (Figure 8.2).

First, consider the case where you take a sample of $n = 5$ from both populations. The expected standard error of the mean will be $\frac{\sigma}{\sqrt{n}} = \frac{1250}{\sqrt{5}} = 559.02$. Therefore, the range around μ within which you would expect 95% of sample means from the **untreated population** to occur would be $\mu \pm 1.96 \times$ SEM, which is $7500 \pm (1.96 \times 559.02)$ and thus 7500 ± 1095.67, giving a range from 6404.33 to 8595.67.

With an effect size of 700, the range around μ (treated) within which you would expect 95% of sample means from the **experimental population** is 8200 ± 1095.67, which is from 7104.33 to 9295.67.

These two ranges are shown in Figure 8.3(a). **Importantly, they overlap considerably, with most of the means of samples from the treated population falling within the expected range of the means of samples from the untreated population.** Therefore, if you were to treat five people with leucoxifen, there is a very high probability that your sample mean from the treatment group will fall within the 95% confidence interval of the **untreated** population and thus would not be considered significantly different to μ. **Even though there is a real effect of this drug, your sample**

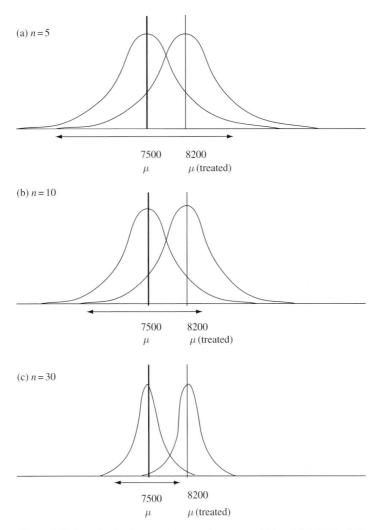

(a) $n = 5$

7500
μ

8200
μ (treated)

(b) $n = 10$

7500
μ

8200
μ (treated)

(c) $n = 30$

7500
μ

8200
μ (treated)

Figure 8.3 Sample size has an effect on the range within which 95% of the means of samples from a population will occur. The expected distributions of the means of samples taken from two populations with the same variance, one of which has a μ of 7500 and the other which has a μ of 8200, are shown. (a) When $n = 5$ the sample means are expected to occur within a relatively wide range around each mean. (b) When $n = 10$ the sample means are expected to occur within a narrower range. (c) When $n = 30$ the sample means are expected to occur within a much narrower range.

size is too small to detect it very often, so you will frequently make a Type 2 error.

Now, consider the case where you have ten people in your experimental group. As sample size increases, the standard error of the mean, and therefore the 95% confidence interval of the mean, will reduce.

For a sample size of ten the standard error of the mean $= \dfrac{\sigma}{\sqrt{n}} = \dfrac{1250}{\sqrt{10}} = 395.3$. Therefore, for samples where $n = 10$, the 95% confidence interval for the distribution of values of the mean around μ is 7500 ± 774.76 (which is from 6725.24 to 8274.76) and the distribution around μ (treated) is 8200 ± 774.76 (which is from 7425.24 to 8974.76). These two ranges are shown in Figure 8.3(b). The confidence intervals have been reduced, but the majority of the sample means from the treated population still lie within the range expected from the untreated population, so the risk of Type 2 error is still very high.

Finally, for a sample size of 30 the standard error will be greatly reduced at $\dfrac{1250}{\sqrt{30}} = 228.22$. Therefore, the 95% confidence interval for the means of sample size 30 will be $\mu \pm 447.3$, which is from 7052.7 to 7947.3 for the untreated population and from 7752.7 to 8647 for the treated population (Figure 8.3(c)). There is less overlap between the 95% confidence intervals of both groups, so you are less likely to make a Type 2 error.

Even when the sample size is 30, there is still a considerable risk of failing to reject the null hypothesis that $\mu = 7500$, because about 25% of the possible values of the sample mean from the treated population are still within the region expected if the mean of 7500 is correct (Figure 8.4).

The probability of Type 2 error is symbolised by β and is **the probability of failing to reject the null hypothesis when it is false**. Therefore, as shown in Figure 8.4, the value of β is the shaded area of the treated distribution lying to the left of the upper confidence interval for μ.

8.4   The power of a test

The power of a test is the probability of making the correct decision and rejecting the null hypothesis when it is false. Therefore power is the area of the treated distribution to the **right** of the vertical line in Figure 8.4. If you know β, you can calculate power as $1 - \beta$.

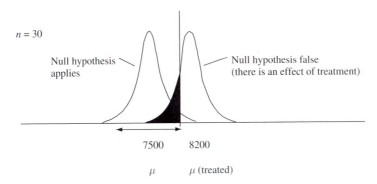

Figure 8.4 The probability of a Type 2 error is the shaded area to the left of the horizontal line marking the upper confidence limit of μ. The risk of Type 2 error is considerable, but it will be even greater if the sample size is smaller.

An 80% power is considered desirable. That is, there is only a 20% chance of a Type 2 error and an 80% chance of **not** making a Type 2 error when the null hypothesis is false.

8.4.1   What determines the power of a test?

The power of a test depends on several things, only some of which can be controlled by the researcher.

The **uncontrollable** factors are **effect size** and the **variance of the population**.

As effect size increases, power will increase and will eventually be 100% as the two distributions get further and further apart (Figure 8.5(a)).

Samples from populations with a relatively small variance will have a smaller standard error of the mean, so overlap between the untreated and treated distributions will be less than for samples from populations with a larger variance (Figure 8.5(b)).

The **controllable** factors are the **sample size** and your **chosen value of** α.

As sample size increases, your risk of Type 2 error decreases and power therefore increases since the standard error of the mean decreases (this has already been described in Figure 8.3).

As the chosen value of α decreases (e.g. from 0.10 to 0.05 to 0.01 to 0.001), the risk of Type 1 error decreases, but the risk of a Type 2 error increases. This is shown in Figure 8.6. There is a trade-off between the risks of Type 1 and Type 2 errors.

(a)

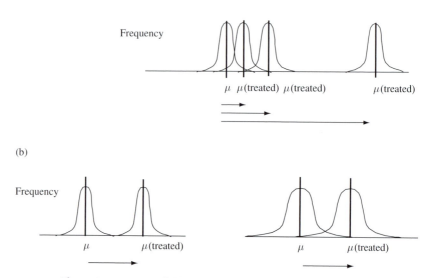

(b)

Figure 8.5 Uncontrollable factors affecting power. (a) Effect size will determine power and, if the effect size is large enough, power will be 100%. The arrows show effect size. (b) With a fixed effect size, a test comparing the distribution of sample means from a population with a relatively small variance (the pair of graphs on the left) will have greater power than if the population variance is large (the pair of graphs on the right).

8.5   What sample size do you need to ensure the risk of Type 2 error is not too high?

Without compromising the risk of Type 1 error, the only way a researcher can reduce the risk of Type 2 error to an acceptable level and therefore ensure sufficient power is to increase their sample size. Every researcher has to ask themselves the question, 'What sample size do I need to ensure the risk of Type 2 error is low and therefore power is high?' This is an important question because samples are usually costly to take, so there is no point in increasing sample size past the point where power reaches an acceptable level. For example, if a sample size of 35 gave 100% power, there is no point in taking a larger sample.

Unfortunately, the only way to estimate the appropriate minimum sample size needed in an experiment is to know, or have good estimates of, the effect size and standard deviation of the population(s). Often the

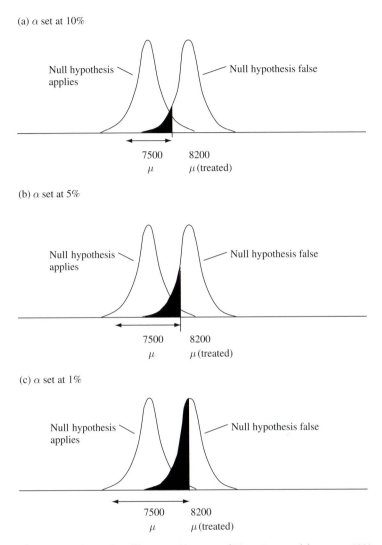

(a) α set at 10%

Null hypothesis applies

Null hypothesis false

7500
μ

8200
μ (treated)

(b) α set at 5%

Null hypothesis applies

Null hypothesis false

7500
μ

8200
μ (treated)

(c) α set at 1%

Null hypothesis applies

Null hypothesis false

7500
μ

8200
μ (treated)

Figure 8.6 The trade-off between Type 1 and Type 2 error. (a) α set at 10%. (b) Decreasing α to 5% will reduce the risk of Type 1 error, but will increase the risk of Type 2 error. (c) Decreasing α to 1% will further decrease the risk of Type 1 error, but greatly increase the risk of Type 2 error.

only way to estimate these is to do a pilot experiment with a sample. For most tests there are formulae that use these (sample) statistics to give the appropriate sized sample for a desired power. Some statistical packages will calculate the power of a test as part of the analysis.

8.6   Type 1 error, Type 2 error, and the concept of biological risk

The commonly used α of 0.05 sets the risk of Type 1 error at 5%, while 20% is considered an acceptable risk of Type 2 error. **Nevertheless, these risks have to be considered in relation to the consequences of an incorrect decision about the null or alternate hypotheses.** There was a discussion about the appropriate risk of Type 1 error depending on the consequences in Chapter 5 and the same considerations apply to the risk of Type 2 error.

For example, a test that has a 20% chance of incorrectly retaining the null hypothesis of no effect may be considered inappropriate if you are testing for the undesirable side effects of a new drug, or evaluating whether the release of sewage into a river is affecting the number of bacteria pathogenic to humans in a lake downstream. Every time you run a statistical test you have to consider not only the risks of Type 1 and Type 2 errors, but also the consequences of these risks.

8.7   Conclusion

Whenever you make a decision based on the probability of a result, there is a risk of either a Type 1 or a Type 2 error. There is only a risk of Type 1 error when the null hypothesis applies, and the risk is the chosen probability level α. There is only a risk of Type 2 error when the null hypothesis is false. Here the risk of Type 2 error, β, is affected by several factors, but the most controllable is sample size. As sample size increases, the risk of Type 2 error decreases.

Power is the converse of Type 2 error. Power is $1 - \beta$ and is the ability of the test to reject the null hypothesis when it is false.

There are formulae for calculating the appropriate sample size to ensure that the risk of Type 2 error is acceptable (e.g. 20%) and thereby have acceptable power, but these calculations rely on an estimate of effect size and the standard deviation of the sample or population.

Finally, the risks of Type 1 and Type 2 errors need to be considered in terms of biological risk – depending on the consequences of making each type of error, you may find an α of 5%, or a β of 20%, unacceptable.

9 | Single factor analysis of variance

9.1 Introduction

So far, this book has only covered tests for one and two samples. Often, however, you are likely to have univariate data from three or more samples, from different locations or experimental groups, and wish to test the hypothesis that, 'The means of the populations from which these samples have come from are not significantly different to each other', or '$\mu_1 = \mu_2 = \mu_3 = \mu_4 = \mu_5$ etc . . . '.

For example, you might have data for the length in millimetres of adult grasshoppers of the same species from five different regions and wish to test the hypothesis that the samples have come from populations with the same mean.

Here you could test this hypothesis by doing a lot of two sample t tests that compare all of the possible pairs of means (e.g. mean 1 compared with mean 2, mean 1 compared with mean 3, mean 2 compared with mean 3 etc.). The problem with this approach is that every time you do a two sample test and the null hypothesis applies you run a 5% risk of a Type 1 error. So, as you do more and more tests on the same set of data, the risk of a Type 1 error rises rapidly.

Put simply, every time you do a two sample test it is like having a ticket in a lottery where the chance of winning is 5% – the more tickets you have, the more likely you are to win. Here, however, to 'win' could be to make the wrong decision about your results. If you have five groups, there are ten possible pairwise comparisons among them and the risk of a getting a Type 1 error when using an α of 0.05 is 40%, which is extremely high (Box 9.1).

Obviously there is a need for a test that compares three or more groups simultaneously, but only has a risk of Type 1 error the same as your chosen value of α. This is where analysis of variance (ANOVA) can often be used.

Box 9.1 The probability of a Type 1 error increases when you make several pairwise comparisons

Every time you do a statistical test where the null hypothesis applies, the risk of a Type 1 error is your chosen value of α. If α is 0.05, then the probability of **not** making a Type 1 error is $(1 - \alpha)$ or 0.95.

If you have three treatment means and therefore make three pairwise comparisons (1 versus 2, 2 versus 3, and 1 versus 3), the probability of **no** Type 1 errors is $(0.95)^3 = 0.86$. The probability of **at least** one Type 1 error is 0.14 or 14%.

For four treatment means there are six possible comparisons, so the probability of **no** Type 1 errors is $(0.95)^6 = 0.74$. The probability of **at least** one Type 1 error is 0.26 or 26%.

For five treatment means there are ten possible comparisons, so the probability of **no** Type 1 error is $(0.95)^{10} = 0.60$. The probability of **at least** one Type 1 error is 0.40 or 40%.

These risks are unacceptably high. You need a test that compares more than two treatment means with a Type 1 error the same as α.

A lot of scientists make decisions on the results of ANOVA without knowing how it works. But it is very important to understand how ANOVA does work so that you can appreciate its uses and limitations!

Analysis of variance was developed by the statistician Sir Ronald A. Fisher from 1918 onwards. It is a very elegant technique and can be applied to numerous and very complex experimental designs. This book introduces the simpler ANOVA models, because an understanding of these makes the more complex ones easier. The following is a pictorial explanation, like the pictorial explanations developed to explain t tests in Chapter 7. This approach is remarkably simple and does represent what happens. By contrast, a look at the equations in many statistics texts makes ANOVA seem very confusing indeed.

9.2   Single factor analysis of variance

Imagine you are interested in assessing the effects of two experimental drugs on the growth of brain tumours in humans. Many of these tumours

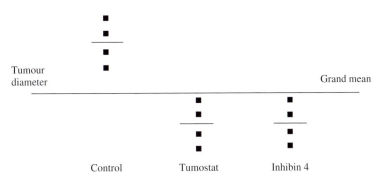

Figure 9.1 Pictorial representation of the diameter of human brain tumours in clinical volunteers either left untreated (control) or treated with the experimental drugs Tumostat or Inhibin 4. Tumour diameter increases up the page. The heavy horizontal line shows the grand mean, while the shorter lighter lines show treatment means. The diameter of each replicate tumour is shown as a filled square ■.

cannot be removed because the brain would be badly damaged in the process. A growing tumour will compress and replace neural tissue, often causing fatal damage, so there is great medical interest in drugs that affect tumour growth.

You have been assigned 12 consenting experimental subjects, each of whom has a brain tumour of the same size and type. Four are allocated at random to an untreated control group, four are treated with the drug 'Tumostat' and four more with the drug 'Inhibin 4'. After two months of treatment, their tumours are remeasured. Your null hypothesis is that, 'There is no difference in mean tumour diameter among the populations from which these three samples have been taken.' The alternate hypothesis is, 'There is a difference in mean tumour diameter among the populations from which these samples have been taken'.

The results of this experiment have been displayed pictorially in Figure 9.1, with tumour diameter (in millimetres) increasing on the Y axis and the three treatment categories on the X axis. The sample means of each group of four are shown, together with the **grand mean**, which is the mean diameter of all 12 tumours.

Now, think about the diameter of each tumour. There are two possible sources of variation that will contribute to its displacement from the grand mean.

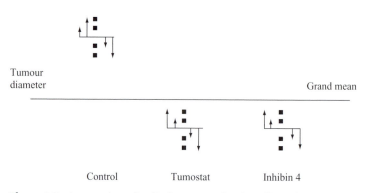

Tumour
diameter   Grand mean

Control   Tumostat   Inhibin 4

Figure 9.2 Arrows show the displacement of each replicate from its
respective treatment mean. This is the variation due to error only.

First, there is the effect of the treatment it has experienced (Control or
Tumostat or Inhibin 4).

Second, there is likely to be variation among individuals that cannot be
controlled, such as slight differences in initial tumour size, differences in
the general health, genotype, nutritional state, and immune responses of
each person, plus other unintended aspects of the experiment, as discussed
in Chapter 3. This uncontrollable variation is called 'error'.

Therefore, the displacement of each point on the Y axis from the grand
mean will be determined by the following formula:

$$\text{Tumour diameter} = \text{treatment} + \text{error} \qquad (9.1)$$

In the example shown in Figure 9.1, Tumostat and Inhibin 4 appear to have
an inhibitory effect on growth compared with the control (in which the
tumours have grown larger) **but is the effect significant, or is it just the
sort of difference that might occur by chance among samples taken from
populations with the same mean?** A single factor ANOVA calculates this
probability in a very straightforward way. The key to understanding how
the ANOVA does this is to consider the reasons why the values for each
tumour and the treatment means are where they are.

First, the diameter of each tumour will be displaced from its treatment
mean by error only. This is called **error** or **within group variation**
(Figure 9.2).

Second, each treatment mean will be displaced from the grand mean by
any effect of that treatment plus error. Here, since we are dealing with

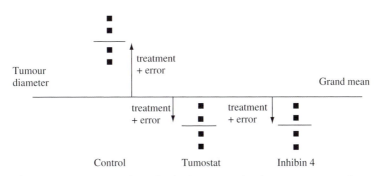

Figure 9.3 The arrows show the displacement of each treatment mean from the grand mean and represent the average effect of the treatment plus error for the replicates in that treatment.

treatment means, the distance between a particular treatment mean and the grand mean is the average effect of all of the replicates within that treatment. To get the total effect you have to think of this displacement occurring for each of the replicates. This is called **among group variation** (Figure 9.3).

Third, the diameter of each tumour will be displaced from the grand mean by **both sources of variation** – the within group variation (Figure 9.2) plus the among group variation (Figure 9.3) described above. This is called the **total variation** in the experiment. In Figure 9.4, the distance displaced is shown for the four tumours in each treatment.

Each of Figures 9.2–9.4 show the dispersion of points around means. Therefore it is possible to calculate a separate variance from each figure.

(a) **The within group variance, which is due to error only** (Figure 9.2), can be calculated from the dispersion of the points around each of their respective treatment means.

(b) **The among group variance, which is due to treatment and error** (Figure 9.3), can be calculated from the dispersion of the treatment means around the grand mean. The distance between each treatment mean and the grand mean will represent the average effect for the number of replicates in that treatment.

(c) **The total variance** (Figure 9.4) is the combined effects of the within group variance and the among group variance (quantities (a) and (b) above). This can be calculated from the dispersion of all the points around the grand mean.

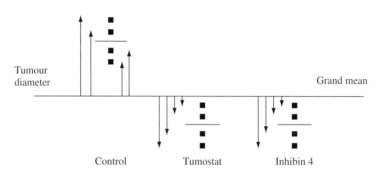

Figure 9.4 Arrows show the displacement of each replicate from the grand mean. The length of each arrow represents the total variation affecting each replicate.

These estimates give a very easy way of assessing whether the three treatment means have come from populations with the same mean μ.

First, if there is no effect of any treatment, the among group variance (due to treatment plus error) will be a small number, because all the treatment means will only be displaced from the grand mean by any effect of error (Figure 9.5(a)).

Second, if there is a relatively large treatment effect, some or all of the treatment means will be very different to each other and further away from the grand mean. Therefore the among group variance (due to treatment plus error) will be large compared with the within group variance (due to error only) (Figure 9.5(b)). As the differences among treatments get larger and larger so will the among group variance.

Therefore, to get a statistic that shows the **relative effect of the treatments compared with error, all you have to do is calculate the among group variance (due to the treatments plus error) and divide this by the within group variance (due to error):**

$$\frac{\text{Among group variance (treatment} + \text{error)}}{\text{Within group variance (error)}} \qquad (9.2)$$

If there is no treatment effect, then both the numerator and denominator of equation (9.2) will only estimate error, so the value of this statistic will be approximately 1.0 (Figure 9.5(a)). But, as the treatment effect increases (Figure 9.5(b)), the numerator of equation (9.2) will get larger and larger, so the value of the statistic will also increase. As it

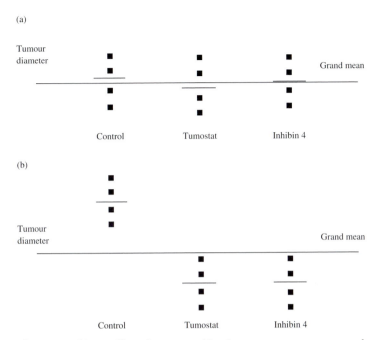

Figure 9.5 (a) No effect of treatment. The three treatment means are only displaced from the grand mean because of error, so the among group variance will be relatively small. (b) An effect of treatment. There are relatively large differences among the treatment means, so they are further from the grand mean, making the among group variance relatively large.

increases, the probability that the treatments have been taken from populations with the same mean will **decrease** and will eventually be less than 0.05.

The statistic obtained by dividing one variance by another was previously mentioned in Section 7.7.3 and is called the **F statistic** or **F ratio**. Once an F ratio is calculated, its significance can be assessed by looking up the expected distribution of F under the null hypothesis of no difference among the treatment means. Just like the example of the chi-square statistic discussed in Chapter 2 and the Z and t statistics in Chapter 7, even when the treatment groups are drawn from populations with the same mean (that is, there is no effect of any of the treatments) the value of the statistic will, just by chance, be larger than a particular value in 5% of cases and be considered statistically significant.

9.3   An arithmetic/pictorial example

Doing a single factor analysis of variance is straightforward and the following example will also help you interpret the results provided by statistics programs.

Here I am using a simple set of data for tumour diameter (in mm) for four replicates of three chosen treatments in another experiment involving two experimental drugs (Table 9.1).

To do a single factor ANOVA, all you have to do is calculate the among group (treatment) variance and divide this by the within group (error) variance to get the F ratio. The procedure is shown pictorially in Figures 9.6–9.9.

9.3.1   Preliminary steps

First, you calculate the grand mean, by taking the sum of all the values, and dividing this by n (which in this example is 12). The value of the grand mean is shown in the large box to the right of the line indicating the position of the grand mean in Figure 9.6.

Second, you calculate each treatment mean, by taking the sum of the values in each treatment and dividing by the appropriate sample size (here, in each case it is 4). These values are shown in the boxes to the right of the lines indicating each treatment mean.

These are all the values you need to calculate the three different variances.

Figures 9.7, 9.8, and 9.9 show the calculation of the total, error, and treatment variances. The general formula for any sample variance is:

$$\sum \frac{(X_i - \bar{X})^2}{n - 1} \tag{9.3}$$

Table 9.1. The diameter of 12 brain tumours in mm after three months of either (a) no treatment, (b) treatment with Neurohib, or (c) treatment with Mitostop

Control	Neurohib	Mitostop
7	4	1
8	5	2
10	7	4
11	8	5

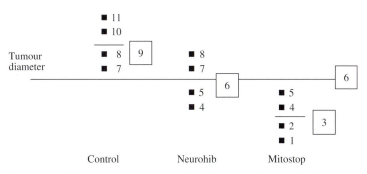

Figure 9.6 Pictorial representation of the diameter of human brain tumours in clinical volunteers either left untreated (control) or treated with the experimental drugs Neurohib or Mitostop. Tumour diameter increases up the page. The heavy horizontal line shows the grand mean, while the shorter lighter lines show treatment means. The tumour diameter of each replicate is shown as ■. Boxes show the values of the treatment means and the grand mean.

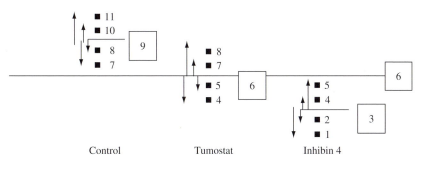

Step 1: The within group (error) **sum of squares** is:

Control					Tumostat					Inhibin 4				Sum of squares
4	1	1	4	+	4	1	1	4	+	4	1	1	4	=	30

Step 2: The within group (error) **variance** is $30 \div 9 = 3.33$

Figure 9.7 Calculation of the within group (error) sum of squares and variance. This has been done in two stages. First, the displacement of each point from its treatment mean has been squared and these values added together to get the sum of squares. Second, the sum of squares has been divided by the number of degrees of freedom to give the mean square, which is the within group (error) variance.

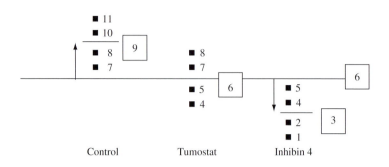

Step 1: The total among group (treatment) **sum of squares** is the sum of the average displacement of each treatment, squared and multiplied by the sample size of each treatment:

Control		Tumostat		Inhibin 4		Sum of squares
9	× 4 +	0	× 4 +	9	× 4 =	72

Step 2: The among group (treatment) **variance** is $72 \div 2 = 36$

Figure 9.8 Calculation of the among group (treatment) sum of squares and variance. This has been done in two steps. First, the displacement of each treatment mean from the grand mean has been squared. This value has to be multiplied by the sample size within each treatment to get the total effect for the replicates within that treatment because the displacement is the average for the treatment. These three values are then added together to give the sum of squares. Second, the sum of squares has been divided by the number of degrees of freedom to give the mean square value, which is the among group (treatment) variance. Note that one of the treatment means happens to be the same as the grand mean, but this will not always occur.

and the variances have been calculated in two steps. First the sum of each value minus the appropriate mean and then squared (the numerator of the equation above which is called the **sum of squares**) has been calculated. Second this value has been divided by the appropriate degrees of freedom (the denominator of the equation above) to give the variance, which is often called the **mean square**.

9.3.2   Calculation of within group variation (error)

This has been done in two steps in Figure 9.7. First, you calculate the sum of squares for error. The distance between each replicate and its treatment

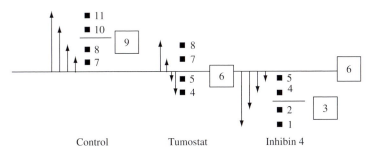

Control   Tumostat   Inhibin 4

Step 1: The total **sum of squares** is:

Control					Tumostat					Inhibin 4				Sum of squares
25	16	4	1	+	4	1	1	4	+	25	16	4	1	=	102

Step 2: There are 11 degrees of freedom, so the total **variance** is $102 \div 11 = 9.273$

Figure 9.9 Calculation of the total sum of squares and total variation. This has been done in two steps. First, the displacement of each point from the grand mean has been squared, and these values added together to give the sum of squares. Second, the sum of squares has been divided by the number of degrees of freedom to give the mean square, which is the total variance.

mean is the error associated with that replicate. You square each of these values and add them together to get the sum of squares.

Second, you calculate the mean square by dividing the total by the number of degrees of freedom. Here you need the sum of the number of replicates in each treatment minus 1. Since each treatment contains four replicates the number of degrees of freedom is $3 + 3 + 3 = 9$.

9.3.3   Calculation of among group variation (treatment)

This has been done in two steps in Figure 9.8.

First, you calculate the sum of squares for treatment. The distance between any of the three treatment means and the grand mean is the average effect of that treatment. Therefore, to get the total effect for all the replicates within each treatment, this value has to be squared **and then multiplied by the number of replicates in that treatment** and these values added together to give the sum of squares for treatment.

Second, you calculate the mean square by dividing the sum of squares by the degrees of freedom, which is $n - 1$ where n is the number of

Table 9.2. Summary of the results of the calculations from Figures 9.7–9.9. The results have been formatted as a typical single factor ANOVA summary table provided by most statistical software packages

Source of variation	Sum of squares	df	Mean square	F ratio	Probability
Among groups (treatment)	72	2	36.0	10.8	0.004
Within groups (error)	30	9	3.3		
Total	102	11			

treatments. Here, since there are three treatments, there are only two degrees of freedom.

9.3.4   Calculation of the total variation

First you calculate the sum of squares for the total variation by taking the displacement of each point from the grand mean, squaring it and adding these together for all replicates. This gives the total sum of squares. Dividing the total sum of squares by the total number of degrees of freedom (there are $n-1$ degrees of freedom, and in this case $n = 12$) gives the mean square. This has been done in two steps in Figure 9.9.

Finally, to obtain the F ratio, which compares the effect of treatment to the effect of error, you simply divide the **among group (treatment) variance** by the **within group (error) variance**.

Since the treatment variance is 36 (Figure 9.8) and the error variance is 3.33 (Figure 9.7), the F ratio of treatment variance /error variance is $36/3.33 = 10.8$. Table 9.2 gives the results of this analysis in a similar format to the one provided by most statistical packages.

Here you may be wondering why the total sum of squares and total variance in the experiment have been calculated, since they are not needed for the F ratio given above. The calculation has been included to illustrate the additivity of the sums of squares and degrees of freedom. Note from Table 9.2 that the total sum of squares (102) is the sum of the treatment (72) plus the error (30) sums of squares. Note also that the total degrees of freedom (11) is the sum of the treatment (2) plus the error (9) degrees of freedom. This additivity of sums of squares and degrees of freedom will be used when discussing more complex ANOVA models.

Now, all you need is the critical value of the F ratio. This used to be a tedious procedure because there are two values of the degrees of freedom to consider – the one associated with the treatment mean square and the one associated with the error mean square – and you had to look up the critical value in a large set of tables. Here, however, you can use a statistics program to run this analysis, generate the F ratio, and obtain the probability. It is shown in the column on the far right of Table 9.2 and is significant since it is less than 0.05.

The F ratio is always written with the number of degrees of freedom for the numerator and denominator given in order as a subscript. Therefore the F ratio for the among group mean square divided by the within group mean square from Table 9.2 would be written as $F_{2,9}$, because there are two degrees of freedom for the among group variance and nine degrees of freedom for the within group variance.

9.4   Unequal sample sizes (unbalanced designs)

The example described above has used an experimental design with equal numbers in each treatment. If they are not equal the method for calculating the F ratio will still work, but the means and variances within each group will not be estimated with the same precision (Chapter 6). For example, the mean of a relatively small sample is likely to be less accurate than that of a larger one, so the conclusion from a comparison of means may be misleading. You should, wherever possible, aim to have equal numbers in each treatment, especially when sample sizes are relatively small.

9.5   An ANOVA does not tell you which particular treatments appear to be from different populations

Although a significant result of a single factor ANOVA indicates that the treatment means are unlikely to come from populations with the same mean, it has not shown where the differences actually lie. In the example given above, a significant effect might be caused by one or both experimental drugs actually enhancing tumour growth compared with the control! You will almost certainly want to know how each of the two drugs actually affect tumour growth. To do this, you will need to make multiple comparisons among the treatment means. This procedure is described in Chapter 10.

9.6 Fixed or random effects

This is an important concept. There are two types of single factor ANOVA models, which are called **Model I** and **Model II**. An understanding of the difference between them is necessary, especially when you meet two factor ANOVAs later in this book.

A Model I or **fixed effects** ANOVA applies when the treatments (e.g. the experimental drugs) have been **specifically chosen**. For example, you are only interested in the effect of a particular set of four drugs and the null hypothesis reflects this – for example, 'There is no difference between the effects of drugs A, B, C, and D on tumour growth.'

A Model II or **random effects** ANOVA applies to more general hypotheses. For example, instead of seeking the effects of specific drugs, the hypothesis is, 'There is no difference among drugs, in general, on tumour growth.' Therefore the drugs chosen and used in the experiment are merely **random representatives** of the wider range of drugs available, even though your random selection might be drugs A, B, C, and D.

For a single factor ANOVA the actual computations for both models are the same. But, if you have done a Model II ANOVA, you would not normally go any further and make multiple comparisons among treatments because you would not be interested in knowing which ones were different. This is discussed in more detail in Chapter 10. When you do two factor ANOVAs, which are discussed in Chapter 11, it also matters whether the effects are fixed or random.

10 | Multiple comparisons after ANOVA

10.1 Introduction

When you use a single factor ANOVA to examine the results of an experiment with three or more treatments, a significant result only indicates that one or more appear to come from populations with different means. **It does not identify which particular treatment means appear to be from the same or different populations.**

For example, a significant difference among the means of the three treatments A, B, and C can occur in several ways. Mean A may be greater (or less) than B and C; mean B may be greater (or less) than A and C; mean C may be greater (or less) than A and B; and, finally, means A, B, and C may all be different to each other.

If the treatments have been chosen as random representatives of all the possible treatments available (i.e. the factor is random so you have done a Model II ANOVA), you will not be interested in knowing which particular treatment means appear to be from the same or different populations because your hypothesis is more general. A significant result will reject the null hypothesis and show a difference, but that is all you will want to know.

In contrast, if the treatments have been specifically chosen (i.e. the factor is fixed so you have done a Model I ANOVA), you will be interested in knowing which treatment means appear to be from the same or different populations. There are several multiple comparison tests designed to do this.

10.2 Multiple comparison tests after a Model I ANOVA

Multiple comparison tests are used to make comparisons among a set of means and assign them to groups that appear to be from the same population. These tests are usually done after a Model I ANOVA has shown a significant difference among treatments. They are called *a posteriori* or *post hoc* tests, both of which mean 'after the event', where the 'event' is a significant result of the ANOVA.

A lot of multiple comparison tests have been developed, but all of them work in essentially the same way. Here is an example using the Tukey test, which works in an analogous way to the two sample t test described in Chapter 7.

The t statistic is calculated by dividing the difference between two means by the standard error of that difference. The Tukey statistic, q, is calculated by dividing the difference between two means by the standard error of the mean. The smaller mean is always taken away from the larger, therefore giving a positive number:

$$q = \frac{\bar{X}_A - \bar{X}_B}{\text{SEM}} \tag{10.1}$$

This procedure is first used to compare the largest mean to the smallest. If the difference is significant, testing continues by comparing the largest with the next smallest and so on. If a non-significant difference is found, all the means included within the range between that pair are assigned to the same population. Then the procedure is repeated, starting with the second largest and the smallest mean; repeated again starting with the third largest and the smallest mean, and so on. Eventually the means will be assigned to one or more groups, each containing those which appear to be from the same population (Figure 10.1).

From the example in Figure 10.1, means A, B, and C appear to be from the same population and D and E from a second population. The analysis has revealed two distinct groups.

For the Tukey statistic you need the SEM and the best way to obtain this is from the error mean square of the ANOVA, because this is an estimate of the population variance, σ^2, calculated from the displacement of all the replicates in the experiment from their respective treatment means. Therefore, since the standard error of a mean is:

$$\text{SEM} = \frac{\sigma}{\sqrt{n}} \quad \text{or} \quad \sqrt{\frac{\sigma^2}{n}} \tag{10.2}$$

the standard error of the mean estimated from an ANOVA is:

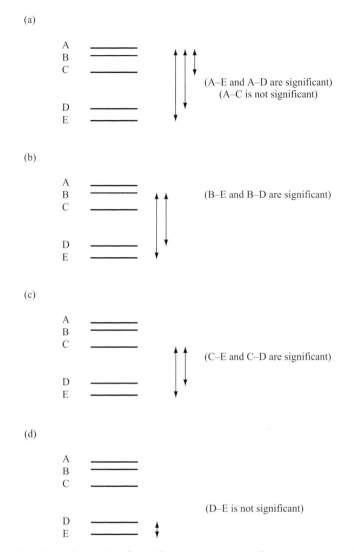

Figure 10.1 General procedure for a Tukey a-posteriori test. The treatment means (A–E) are displayed in order of magnitude from the smallest (E) to the largest (A). (a) First the largest mean is compared with the smallest (A–E). If the difference is significant, the largest is then compared with the second smallest (A–D) and so on, until a non-significant difference (here, as an example, A–C) is found or there are no more pairs of means left to compare. All means included within the range between A–C (A, B, and C) are assigned to the same population. (b) Testing continues using the same procedure but starting with the second largest mean and comparing it with the smallest (B–E). (c) The third largest mean (C) is compared with D and E. (d) The fourth largest (D) is compared with E. This difference is not significant so D and E appear to be from the same population, which has a different mean to the one from which A, B, and C have been taken.

$$\text{SEM} = \sqrt{\frac{\text{MS error}}{n}} \qquad (10.3)$$

where n is the sample size of each treatment. If the treatment sample sizes are different, you use the formula:

$$\text{SEM} = \sqrt{\frac{\text{MS error}}{2} \times \left(\frac{1}{n_A} + \frac{1}{n_B}\right)} \qquad (10.4)$$

Then you calculate the Tukey statistic q for each pair of means by using equation (10.1) and the procedure in Figure 10.1.

The calculated value of q will be zero when there is no difference between the two sample means and will increase as the difference between the means increases. If q exceeds the critical value, the hypothesis that the means are from the same population is rejected.

The critical value of q depends upon your chosen value of α, the number of degrees of freedom for the MS error, and the number of means being tested. Here I deliberately have not given a table of q values because most statistical packages will do multiple comparisons and even generate a display assigning the sample means to groups that appear to be from the same population. Section 10.3 gives two examples and also illustrates that ambiguous results are possible.

10.3 An a-posteriori Tukey comparison following a significant result for a single factor Model I ANOVA

10.3.1 The effects of dietary supplements on pig growth

These data are for the amount of weight gained in kilograms by piglets of the same age and initial weight after six months of feeding with four different dietary supplements: 'Pigout', 'Sowgrow', 'Baconbuster II', and 'Fatboar III'. This is a Model I ANOVA – the researcher is only interested in the effects of these four supplements on pig growth.

If you run a single factor ANOVA on the data in Table 10.1, you will obtain an F ratio ($F_{3,16}$) of 74.01, which has a probability of less than 0.001. Some of the treatment means appear to be from different populations. If you then run an a-posteriori Tukey test, you will find that each of the four means appear to be from different populations.

Table 10.1. The weight gain of piglets fed four different dietary supplements

	Pigout	Sowgrow	Baconbuster II	Fatboar III
	16	19	25	12
	14	20	30	10
	16	22	26	12
	17	20	27	13
	18	24	28	9
$\bar{X}$	16.2	21.0	27.2	11.2

10.3.2 Growth of brain tumours treated with experimental drugs

Table 10.2 gives data for the diameter of brain tumours exposed to three months of (a) no treatment (control) or two experimental drugs.

A one factor ANOVA will give an F ratio ($F_{2,9}$) of 10.8, which has a probability of 0.004. The three treatment means do not appear to be from the same population.

If, however, you run an a-posteriori Tukey test, it will show that means for the control and Neurohib appear to be from the same population, while the means for Neurohib and Mitostop appear to be from another.

The result in Figure 10.2 is obviously ambiguous. The a-posteriori analysis has separated the data into two subsets, but the mean of the Neurohib treatment cannot be distinguished from the means of either the control or the Mitostop treatment. At the same time, the mean of the control can be distinguished from the mean for Mitostop. Therefore, it seems a Type 2 error has been committed somewhere, since the mean of the Neurohib treatment has been assigned to two different populations.

10.4   Other a-posteriori multiple comparison tests

There are many other multiple comparison tests. These include the LSD, Bonferroni, Scheffé, and Student–Newman–Keuls. The most commonly used are the Tukey and Student–Newman–Keuls (Zar, 1999). Most statistical packages offer you a wide choice of these tests and their relative merits are described in more advanced texts.

Table 10.2. The diameter of 12 brain tumours in millimetres after three months of either (a) no treatment, (b) treatment with Neurohib, or (c) Mitostop

	Control	Neurohib	Mitostop
	7	4	1
	8	5	2
	10	7	4
	11	8	5
$\bar{X}$	9.0	6.0	3.0

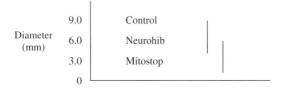

Figure 10.2 Summary of the results of an a-posteriori Tukey test comparing among the means of the three samples in Table 10.2. Treatment means connected by vertical lines are not significantly different.

10.5   Planned comparisons

Chapter 9 began with a discussion about the danger of an increased probability of Type 1 error when making numerous pairwise comparisons among three or more means. Here, however, the a-posteriori method for identifying which treatment means appear to be from the same population uses numerous pairwise comparisons. Therefore, you may well be thinking that this procedure will also have an increased risk of Type 1 error.

First, however, unplanned a-posteriori comparisons are usually only made across all groups if the ANOVA has detected a significant difference among the treatment means. Second, a-posteriori tests are specifically designed to take into account the number of means being compared and have a much lower risk of Type 1 error than the same number of t tests. Unfortunately this makes multiple comparison tests relatively low in power. For example, it sometimes happens that an ANOVA detects a significant difference among treatments, but subsequent a-posteriori testing fails to detect a significant difference among any means.

Instead of making a large number of indiscriminate unplanned a-posteriori comparisons, a better approach can be to make a small number of planned (*a-priori* meaning 'before the event') comparisons. For example, your hypotheses might be that each of the two experimental drugs used in Example 2 above will **reduce** the growth of brain tumours compared with the control. An ANOVA will test for differences among treatments with an α of 0.05 and also give a good estimate of the sample variance from the MS error, since this has been calculated from all the individuals used in the experiment. Next, however, instead of making a large number of unplanned comparisons, you could carry out two (one-tailed) t tests comparing the mean growth of tumours in each drug treatment and the control.

If you make only one planned comparison, the probability of Type 1 error is an acceptable 0.05. If you make several a-priori comparisons that **really have been planned for particular reasons before the experiment** (e.g. to test the hypotheses, 'Mitostop will reduce tumour growth compared to the untreated control' and 'Neurohib will reduce tumour growth compared to the untreated control'), then each is a distinct and different hypothesis, so the risk of a Type 1 error is still an acceptable 0.05. It is only when you make indiscriminate comparisons that the risk of Type 1 error increases and you should consider using one of the a-posteriori tests described previously, which maintains an α of 0.05.

To make a planned comparison after a one factor ANOVA you use the formula for a t test from Chapter 7 except that you use the mean square error as the best estimate of s^2:

$$t_{nA+nB-2} = \frac{\bar{X}_A - \bar{X}_B}{\sqrt{\frac{\text{MS error}}{1} \times \left(\frac{1}{n_A} + \frac{1}{n_B}\right)}} \tag{10.5}$$

which reduces to equation (10.6) when there are equal numbers in both treatment groups:

$$t_{nA+nB-2} = \frac{\bar{X}_A - \bar{X}_B}{\sqrt{\frac{2 \times \text{MS error}}{n}}} \tag{10.6}$$

Here is an example, using the data from Example 2 in Section 10.3. The planned comparison is of the mean tumour size in the Mitostop treatment compared with the control.

From the ANOVA the mean square for error is 3.333. The mean of the Mitostop treatment is 3.0 mm and the control is 9.0 mm. Therefore:

$$t_6 = \frac{3.00 - 9.00}{\sqrt{\frac{2 \times 3.33}{4}}} = -4.65$$

From Table 7.1 the critical one-tailed 5% value for t is 1.943. The two means appear to be from different populations.

Interestingly, the planned comparison to test the effect of Neurohib compared with the control is:

$$t_6 = \frac{6.00 - 9.00}{\sqrt{\frac{2 \times 3.33}{4}}} = -2.325$$

Again, since the critical one-tailed 5% value for t is 1.943, these two means also appear to be from different populations. This example illustrates the value of planned comparisons. Each drug appears to suppress tumour growth compared with the control.

11 | Two factor analysis of variance

11.1   Introduction

A single factor ANOVA gives the probability that two or more sample means have come from populations with the same mean (Chapter 9). Single factor ANOVA is used to analyse univariate data from samples exposed to different levels or aspects of only **one factor**. For example, it could be used to compare the oxygen consumption of a species of intertidal crab (the variable) at two or more temperatures (the factor), the growth of brain tumours (the variable) exposed to a range of drugs (the factor), or the insecticide resistance of a moth (the variable) from several different locations (the factor).

Often, however, life scientists obtain univariate data in relation to **more than one factor**. Examples of two factor experiments are the oxygen consumption of an intertidal crab at several combinations of temperature **and** humidity, the growth of brain tumours exposed to a range of drugs **and** different levels of radiation therapy, or the insecticide resistance of an agricultural pest from different locations **and** different host plants.

It would be very useful to have an analysis that gave separate F ratios (and the probability that the treatment means had come from populations with the same mean) **for each of the two factors**. That is what two factor ANOVA does.

11.1.1 Why do an experiment with more than one factor?

Experiments that simultaneously include the effects of more than one factor on a particular variable may be far more revealing than looking at each factor separately because you may detect certain combinations of factors that have a **synergistic effect**. Also, by examining several factors at once, there may be significant savings in time and resources compared with doing a series of separate experiments and separate analyses.

Table 11.1. Example of an orthogonal two factor design. There are three levels of Factor A (temperature) and two levels of Factor B (humidity) with experimental units (cockroaches) in each of the six possible combinations of the 3 × 2 treatment levels

	Temperature (°C)		
Humidity (%)	20	30	40
33	20 cockroaches	20 cockroaches	20 cockroaches
66	20 cockroaches	20 cockroaches	20 cockroaches

Here is an example of the advantage of a two factor experiment. It also illustrates a synergistic effect – what statisticians call **interaction** – which occurs when the effect of one factor varies across the levels of the other.

Cockroaches are a serious public health risk, especially in tropical and subtropical cities with poor sanitation. These insects often live in sewers and drains, but forage widely and frequently infest areas where food is stored and prepared. Urban cockroaches have a broad diet, which often includes excrement and other wastes, so they can contaminate food and thereby cause disease in humans. An urban entomologist investigating ways of controlling cockroaches was interested in the effects of both temperature and humidity on the activity of the cockroach *Periplaneta americana*. The entomologist devised a method of measuring cockroach activity by placing these insects individually in open topped cylindrical glass jars. By videotaping them from above, and analysing the recordings by computer, the entomologist obtained data for the amount of movement of each cockroach per hour.

The entomologist set up an experiment where cockroaches were kept individually in glass jars in all six combinations of three temperatures (20, 30, and 40°C) and two humidity levels (33 and 66%). There were 20 cockroaches in each treatment, so 120 were used altogether. After two hours of acclimation, activity was recorded for one hour.

This type of design, where there is a treatment for every combination of the levels of each factor used, is called a 'fully orthogonal' design or an 'orthogonal' design (Table 11.1). If one of the treatments were not included (for example the combination of 33% humidity with 20°C), the design would not be orthogonal.

The results of the experiment can be displayed as a graph of the means for each of the six combinations (which are often called **cell means**), with temperature on the X axis, cockroach activity on the Y axis, and lines joining the three means within each of the two levels of humidity. (If you wanted you could show humidity on the X axis and have lines joining each of the three temperatures, but it is easier to visualise when the greatest number of treatment levels are on the X axis.)

Figure 11.1(a) shows a set of cell means where there is **no interaction** – the change in humidity from 33 to 66% (or from 66 to 33%) has the same effect on movement at each temperature (in all cases an increase in humidity increases activity by about the same amount). Similarly, the effect of an increase in temperature from 20°C through to 40°C (or vice versa) is the same at each humidity.

In contrast, Figure 11.1(b) shows **interaction.** A change in humidity from 33 to 66% does not have the same effect on activity at each of the three temperatures, and a change in temperature from 20°C through to 40°C does not have the same effect on activity at each humidity.

That is all interaction is. When there is a complete lack of interaction (e.g. Figure 11.1(a)) the lines joining the treatment means always run exactly parallel to each other (even though both lines move up, they move up in parallel). In contrast, when there is interaction (e.g. Figure 11.1(b)) the lines are not always parallel. As the amount of interaction increases, the lines become less and less parallel and eventually the amount of interaction may reach a point where it is considered significant.

Interaction between two or more factors is often of great interest to life scientists. It may be very helpful to know that a response to one factor is not uniform across the range of a second factor, or that it **is** uniform! For example, if you found that cockroaches are only extremely active when both humidity and temperature are high (Figure 11.1(b)), you might save considerable resources and time by only implementing cockroach control measures when this combination of weather conditions was forecast.

11.2 What does a two factor ANOVA do?

Here you need to remember that a single factor ANOVA partitions the total variation into two components – the variation among groups (treatment + error) and the variation within groups (error) – and examines whether there is a significant effect of treatment by dividing the among groups mean square by the within groups mean square. This gives an

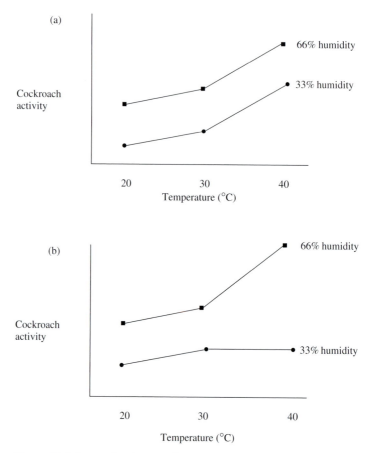

Figure 11.1 Interaction in a two factor experiment. (a) No interaction between the two factors of temperature and humidity on the activity of cockroaches. A change in humidity from 33 to 66% has the same effect on cockroach activity at each of the three temperatures, and a change in temperature from 20°C through to 40°C has the same effect at each humidity. (b) An interaction between temperature and humidity on the activity of cockroaches. A change in humidity from 33 to 66% does not have the same effect on activity at each of the three temperatures, and a change in temperature from 20°C through to 40°C does not have the same effect on activity at each humidity.

F ratio and probability that all the treatment means have come from populations with the same mean.

A two factor ANOVA works in a similar way, but partitions the total variation within a set of data into **four** components: the among group variation due to (a) Factor A + error, (b) Factor B + error, (c) Interaction + error, and (d) error.

The way the analysis works is a straightforward extension of the concept developed to explain single factor ANOVA, and can also be explained pictorially. I will use the simplest case of a two factor design with two levels only of each factor, both of which are fixed.

First, here are some examples of the types of outcomes you might get from a two factor experiment. The urban entomologist mentioned above was also interested in the effects of temperature and humidity on the growth of cockroaches. They did a growth experiment with four newly hatched cockroaches in each treatment, using 16 altogether. Each cockroach was the same starting weight. They were kept at four combinations of two temperatures and two humidities, offered food to excess, and reweighed after four weeks.

Several different outcomes are shown in Figure 11.2. The mean weight gain within each treatment combination of the cockroaches kept at 66% humidity are indicated by ■, while those kept at 33% humidity are indicated by ●.

11.3   How does a two factor ANOVA analyse these data?

This explanation assumes you are familiar with the one already given for a single factor ANOVA in Chapter 9. I am using a two factor experiment with two levels of each factor, giving four treatment combinations, each of which contains four replicates. The design is summarised in Table 11.2. Both factors are fixed – the researcher is only interested in these specific temperatures and humidities.

To start, think about the final weight of each cockroach. It will be displaced from the grand mean by four sources of variation – that associated with **Factor A, plus Factor B, plus interaction, plus error.** This is called the **total variation** in the experiment. Put formally, the position on the Y axis of each replicate in relation to the grand mean will be determined by the following formula:

$$\text{Growth} = \text{Factor A} + \text{Factor B} + \text{interaction} + \text{error} \qquad (11.1)$$

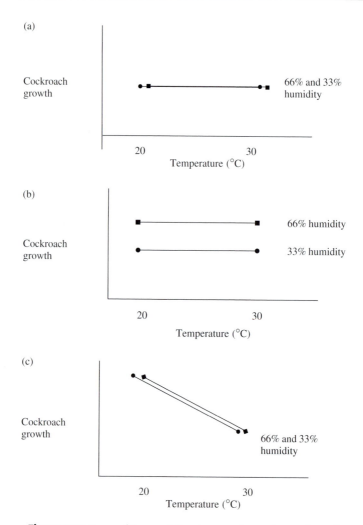

Figure 11.2 Some of the possible outcomes of an orthogonal two factor experiment. (a) No effect of temperature or humidity and no interaction. All treatment means are the same and the lines joining the means within each humidity are also the same. (b) An effect of humidity but no effect of temperature and no interaction. The two treatment means for 66% humidity are consistently more than the two for 33% humidity. (c) An effect of temperature but no effect of humidity and no interaction. The two treatment means for 20°C are consistently greater than the two for 30°C. (d) An effect of temperature and humidity but no interaction. All treatment means are different, but the change in growth in relation to a change in humidity from 33 to 66% is the same at each temperature and vice versa. (e) An effect of temperature and

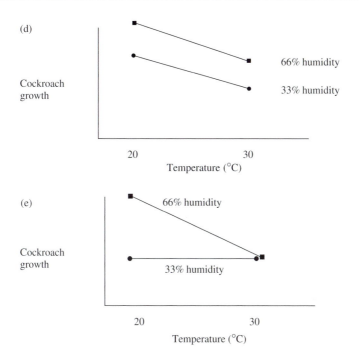

(d)

Cockroach growth

66% humidity

33% humidity

20   30

Temperature (°C)

(e)

Cockroach growth

66% humidity

33% humidity

20   30

Temperature (°C)

Figure 11.2 (cont.) humidity and some interaction. The change in growth from 66 to 33% humidity is not the same at each temperature and vice versa. Only the means for each treatment combination are shown. Note that all lines joining the treatments within the same humidity are parallel except for example (e) where there is some interaction between temperature and humidity.

Table 11.2. The orthogonal design used to explain how two factor ANOVA works in Figures 11.3–11.7. There are four combinations of the two temperatures and two humidities, with four experimental units (cockroaches) in each

Humidity (%)	Temperature (°C)	
	20	30
33	4 cockroaches	4 cockroaches
66	4 cockroaches	4 cockroaches

Here you may wish to contrast this with the much simpler equation for the total variation within a single factor experiment from Chapter 9:

$$\text{Tumour diameter} = \text{treatment} + \text{error} \quad (11.2) \text{ copied from } (9.1)$$

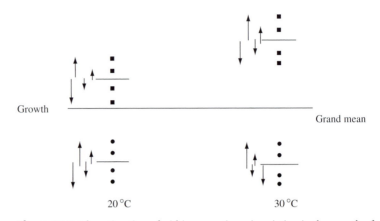

Figure 11.3 The estimation of within group (error) variation in the growth of cockroaches exposed to four different combinations of temperature and humidity. Each cockroach is shown as a symbol: ■ = cockroaches at 66% humidity, ● = cockroaches at 33% humidity. Horizontal lines indicate the grand mean and each cell mean. The displacement of each replicate from its cell mean (arrows) will be caused by error only.

Just as in the single factor ANOVA, the variation within a two factor experiment can be partitioned into several additive components. These are shown in Figures 11.3–11.6.

First, the final weight of each cockroach will be displaced from its respective cell mean by error only. This is estimated in just the same way as for a single factor ANOVA and also called the **within group variation or error** (Figure 11.3). The distances between each replicate and its cell mean are squared and added together to give the within group (error) sum of squares. The sum of squares is divided by the appropriate degrees of freedom (here there are $3 + 3 + 3 + 3 = 12$) to give the within group (error) mean square.

Second, each replicate will be displaced from the grand mean by **all sources of variation in the experiment** – the effect of Factor A, plus Factor B, plus interaction, plus error. This is called the **total variation** in the experiment. In Figure 11.4 below the distance displaced is shown for all replicates. These distances can be squared and added together to give the total sum of squares for the experiment. (Again, this is the same as the procedure for a single factor ANOVA.)

So far, this is the same procedure used to calculate the within group (error) variance and total variance for a single factor ANOVA.

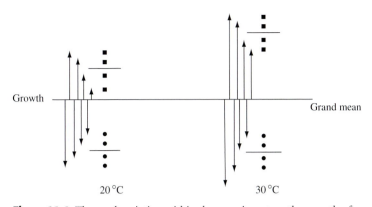

Figure 11.4 The total variation within the experiment on the growth of cockroaches. Each cockroach is shown as a symbol: ■ = cockroaches at 66% humidity, ● = cockroaches at 33% humidity. The heavy horizontal line indicates the grand mean. The four shorter horizontal lines indicate each cell mean. The displacement of each replicate from the grand mean (arrows) will be caused by the total variation within the experiment.

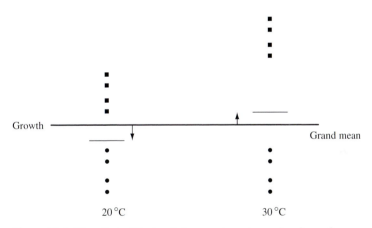

Figure 11.5 The effect of Factor A (temperature + error) only on the growth of cockroaches. Each cockroach is shown as a symbol: ■ = cockroaches at 66% humidity, ● = cockroaches at 33% humidity. These data have been pooled for each temperature, ignoring humidity, thereby generating two new treatment means, shown by the horizontal lines. The displacement of each treatment mean from the grand mean is an estimate of the average effect of temperature plus error. The sum of squares is the sum of each displacement squared, which is then multiplied by the number of replicates in that treatment. The mean square is the sum of squares divided by $n-1$ degrees of freedom, where n is the number of pooled treatments (here $n=2$).

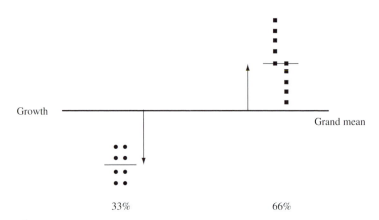

Figure 11.6 The effect of Factor B (humidity + error) only on the growth of cockroaches. Each cockroach is shown as a symbol: ■ = cockroaches at 66% humidity, • = cockroaches at 33% humidity. These data have been pooled for each humidity, ignoring temperature, thereby generating two different treatment means, shown by the horizontal lines. The displacement of each treatment mean from the grand mean is the average effect of humidity for the number of replicates in that treatment. The sum of squares for the effect of humidity is the sum of each displacement squared and multiplied by the number of replicates in that treatment. The mean square is the sum of squares divided by $n - 1$ degrees of freedom, where n is the number of pooled treatments (here $n = 2$).

(a) **The within group variance** (Figure 11.3), which is due to error only, can be calculated from the dispersion of the points around each of their respective cell means.

(b) **The total variance** (Figure 11.4) will estimate the total variation in the experiment (the within group (error) variance, plus Factor A, Factor B, plus interaction), and can be calculated from the dispersion of all the points around the grand mean.

At this stage you still need **separate** effects for Factor A (temperature + error), Factor B (humidity + error), and A × B (interaction + error).

11.4   How does a two factor ANOVA separate out the effects of each factor and interaction?

Two factor ANOVA separates out the effects of each factor and interaction in a very elegant way.

After having done the preliminary calculations in Figures 11.3 to 11.4, the data are only considered in relation to each of the two factors. This is done by first ignoring the different levels within Factor B and considering the data only in relation to Factor A (temperature), after which the same is done for Factor B (humidity). These procedures are shown in Figures 11.5 and 11.6 and allow you to calculate separate sums of squares for temperature + error and also humidity + error. They are called the **simple main effects** because they examine each factor in isolation from the other.

First, the levels of humidity are ignored and the data treated as though they are the results of a single factor experiment on temperature only. Here, therefore, you will have eight replicates within each of the two levels of temperature and you can calculate a mean for each group. These new means, calculated from all eight replicates within each treatment, **will only be displaced from the grand mean by the average effect of temperature plus error**. Therefore, the displacement of the treatment means from the grand mean can be used to calculate the sum of squares and mean square for Factor A (temperature) only (Figure 11.5) just as in a single factor ANOVA.

Second, the levels of temperature are ignored and the data are treated as though they are the results of a single factor experiment on humidity only. Here too, you will have eight replicates within each of the two levels of humidity and you can calculate a mean for each of the two groups. These new means, calculated from all eight replicates within each treatment, **will only be displaced from the grand mean by the average effect of humidity plus error** (Figure 11.6). Therefore, the displacement of the treatment means from the grand mean can be used to calculate the sum of squares and mean square for Factor B (humidity) only, just as in a single factor ANOVA.

At this stage you have sums of squares for the following:

(a) **The total variation in the experiment** (the combined effects of Factor A, Factor B, A × B and error) (Figure 11.4)
(b) **The effect of Factor A** (temperature + error) (Figure 11.5)
(c) **The effect of Factor B** (humidity + error) (Figure 11.6)
(d) **Error** (Figure 11.3)

From this list, the only separate sum of squares you still need is the one for **interaction plus error**. Since the sums of squares are additive and the total variation is the combined effects of all the factors in the ANOVA

Table 11.3. Variation estimated by each mean square term and the appropriate division to estimate the effect of each factor when Factor A and Factor B are both fixed

Source of variation	Calculation of F ratio
Factor A	$\dfrac{\text{Mean square for Factor A}}{\text{Mean square error}}$
Factor B	$\dfrac{\text{Mean square for Factor B}}{\text{Mean square error}}$
Interaction $(A \times B)$	$\dfrac{\text{Mean square for interaction}}{\text{Mean square error}}$

(Section 9.3.4), you can calculate the sum of squares for interaction by subtraction. This is done by taking away the sums of squares for Factor A, Factor B, and error from the total sum of squares ((a) above, minus (b) and (c) and (d)). Now you have the following sums of squares:

- **The total variation in the experiment** (the combined effects of Factor A, Factor B, A × B, and error) (Figure 11.4)
- **The effect of Factor A** (temperature + error) (Figure 11.5)
- **The effect of Factor B** (humidity + error) (Figure 11.6)
- **The effect of interaction** (interaction + error) (by subtraction)
- **Error** (Figure 11.3)

Once you have these, dividing by the appropriate degrees of freedom will give you mean square values, just as for a single factor ANOVA. The effect of each factor can be estimated by dividing the factor mean square by the error mean square to get an F ratio. If the F ratio is significant, the factor is considered to have an effect.

The F ratios for the effects of interaction, Factor A, and Factor B are summarised in Table 11.3.

Most statistical packages will give an analysis of variance summary table that has all of these sums of squares, degrees of freedom, mean square values, and F ratios.

11.5   An example of a two factor analysis of variance

The data in Table 11.4 are for the growth of cockroaches at three temperatures and three levels of humidity.

As an initial step you might plot the cell means on a graph similar to
Figure 11.2 to see what they look like. Which factors might you expect to be
significant? Would you expect a significant interaction? Why?

Next, if you use a statistical package to run a two factor ANOVA on these
data, your results will include something similar to that shown in Table 11.5,
where the F ratio and probability for each of the two factors and their
interaction are given. The interaction term is symbolised by Temperature[*]
Humidity. Note that the F ratios for temperature and humidity are significant at $P < 0.001$, but there is no significant interaction ($P = 0.852$). It

Table 11.4. Length in mm for 27 cockroaches fed ad libitum and
kept in nine different combinations of temperature and humidity

| Temperature (°C) | 20 | 30 | 40 |
Humidity (%)	(level 1)	(level 2)	(level 3)
33 (level 1)	1	5	9
	2	6	10
	3	7	11
66 (level 2)	9	13	17
	10	14	18
	11	15	19
99 (level 3)	17	21	25
	18	22	26
	19	23	27

Table 11.5. An example of the type of output given by a statistical package
for a two factor ANOVA

Source of variation	Sum of squares	df	Mean square	F ratio	Significance
Temperature	312.66	2	156.33	156.33	0.000
Humidity	1200.66	2	600.33	600.33	0.000
Temperature[*] Humidity	1.33	4	0.33	0.33	0.852
Error	18.00	18	1.00		

seems the samples have come from different populations in relation to the levels of temperature and also humidity, but there is no interaction between these factors. This result should not be a surprise if you have plotted the nine treatment means before doing the analysis.

11.6   Some essential cautions and important complications

There are some essential cautions and important complications associated with two factor and more complex ANOVAs that you must be aware of.

1 A significant effect of a factor does not reveal where differences occur if you have examined more than two levels of that factor.
2 A significant interaction can make the F ratios for Factor A or Factor B misleading.
3 If one or both of the factors are random, you need to use a different procedure for calculating the F ratios for one or both of Factors A and B.

These three complications are explained below.

11.6.1   A-posteriori testing is still needed when there is a significant effect of a fixed factor

First, just as for a single factor ANOVA, a significant effect does not reveal where differences occur among the levels of that factor. For example, if you did a two factor ANOVA with four levels of Factor A and six of Factor B, and found a significant effect of Factor A, it will not identify which levels of Factor A appear to come from populations with the same, or different, means. Here, just as for a single factor analysis, you need to carry out a-posteriori testing. This is straightforward if there is no significant interaction.

If the interaction is not significant, a-posteriori testing can be done for each factor that has a significant effect. This compares the mean values for the pooled data (e.g. Figures 11.5 and 11.6) in just the same way as a single factor ANOVA (Chapter 10). For example, if you were to use a Tukey test, the formula is the same as the one given in Chapter 10:

$$q = \frac{\bar{X}_A - \bar{X}_B}{\text{SEM}} \qquad\qquad (11.3)$$

To calculate the standard error of the mean from the ANOVA statistics you use:

$$\text{SEM} = \sqrt{\frac{\text{MS error}}{n}} \tag{11.4}$$

where n is the sample size of each pooled group. If the sample sizes are different, you need to use a slight modification of the formula (which reduces to the one above when n_A is the same size as n_B).

$$\text{SEM} = \sqrt{\frac{\text{MS error}}{2} \times \left(\frac{1}{n_A} + \frac{1}{n_B}\right)} \tag{11.5}$$

Then you simply calculate the Tukey q statistic for each pair of means and look up the critical value of q using the degrees of freedom for MS within groups (error). If the calculated q value is greater than the critical value of q, the hypothesis that the means are from the same population is rejected. The value of q will range from zero when the two sample means are the same, to high values as the means become increasingly different. Once again, many statistical packages will do Tukey tests and assign the means to groups that are significantly different to each other.

Just as with a one factor experiment, a-priori planned comparisons can also be made between particular cell means, but only if these have been specified beforehand (see Section 10.5).

11.6.2 An interaction can obscure a main effect

The two factor analysis described in Section 11.5 gave mean squares for the main effects of Factor A (temperature) and Factor B (humidity), interaction, and also error. The effect of each factor is estimated by dividing the factor mean square by the error mean square.

This is appropriate, but there can be a complication. A significant interaction means that the effect of one factor (e.g. humidity) is not constant across the levels of the second factor (e.g. temperature). **Therefore, if there is a significant interaction, the conclusion of a non-significant main effect (because of a non-significant F ratio for that factor) may not be correct.**

Here is a rather extreme example which clearly illustrates the problem. Imagine an experiment designed to investigate the effects of two treatments, with three levels of Factor A and two of Factor B. Figure 11.7 shows the results of this experiment. Although there is obviously an effect of temperature and also humidity on cockroach activity, the response to temperature at 66% humidity is the opposite of that at 33% humidity.

When these results are analysed by a two factor ANOVA the total sum of squares will be large because the replicates will be well dispersed from the grand mean (Figure 11.7(a)). There will also be some error because the replicates are dispersed from their treatment means (Figure 11.7(a)). But when the ANOVA partitions the sums of squares among the separate factors of temperature and humidity, the results are extremely misleading.

First, consider the pooled analysis for temperature. The new cell means for each of the three levels of temperature (ignoring humidity) will all lie on the grand mean. Consequently there will be **no overall effect of temperature and the sum of squares for temperature will be zero** (Figure 11.7(b)), even though there is obviously an effect of temperature within each level of humidity.

Second, consider the pooled analysis for the two levels of humidity. The new cell means for each of the two levels of humidity (ignoring temperature) will also lie on the grand mean, so the sum of squares for humidity will also be zero (Figure 11.7(c)), even though there is an effect of humidity within each temperature.

The sum of squares for interaction will be realistic and very large.

Therefore, when there is a significant interaction, it is not appropriate to trust the *F* ratios for the effects of Factors A and B. This caution is particularly important because most statistical packages calculate *F* ratios for main effects regardless of whether the interaction is significant or not.

The solution to this problem is straightforward.

A graph of the cell means such as Figure 11.7(a) is a useful first step, because it will give you a visual indication of the positions of each cell mean.

The next step is statistical – you need to look at the effects of each factor across all levels of the second factor using an a-posteriori test. This procedure is a little fiddly, but quite easy to do. Here, shown pictorially, is how you can analyse the cockroach example.

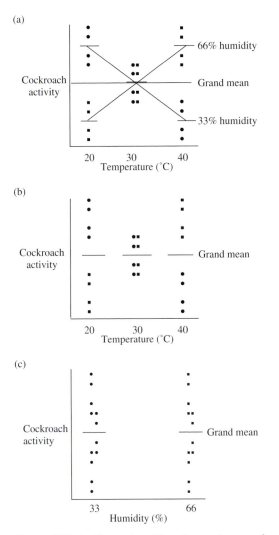

Figure 11.7 An illustration of how interaction can obscure main effects in a two factor ANOVA. (a) As temperature increases, activity decreases at 33% humidity, but increases at 66% humidity. (b) When humidity is ignored the cell means for the three levels of temperature only, are shown as short horizontal lines. Note they all lie on the grand mean. The sum of squares for temperature will be zero. (c) When temperature is ignored the cell means for the two levels of humidity only, are shown as two short horizontal lines. Note they both lie on the grand mean. The sum of squares for humidity will be zero.

(a)

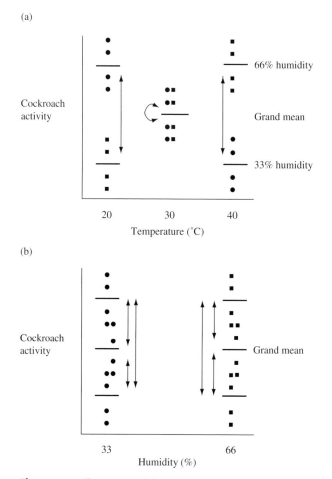

(b)

Figure 11.8 Illustration of the comparisons required for full a-posteriori testing of a two factor ANOVA when there is a significant interaction. (a) Double-headed arrows show the means for the two levels of Factor B (humidity) within each level of Factor A (temperature) compared as part of full a-posteriori testing. (b) Double-headed arrows show the means for the three levels of Factor A (temperature) within each level of Factor B (humidity) compared as part of full a-posteriori testing.

First you compare the two cell means within each of the three levels of temperature (Figure 11.8(a)). Second, you compare the three cell means within each level of humidity (Figure 11.8(b)).

Here too, for a Tukey test, you simply use the formulae:

$$q = \frac{\bar{X}_A - \bar{X}_B}{\text{SEM}} \qquad\qquad (11.5) \text{ copied from } (11.2)$$

and

$$\text{SEM} = \sqrt{\frac{\text{MS error}}{n}} \qquad\qquad (11.6) \text{ copied from } (11.3)$$

where n is the sample size within each cell. Again, the modification to the formula shown in equation (11.7) applies if there are different numbers in each cell.

This rather long but extremely important example emphasises that when there is a significant interaction you need to examine all possible combinations of treatments and that conclusions from F ratios for main effects may not hold.

Most statistical programs will not calculate a-posteriori tests for all possible combinations of cell means given above, so it may be necessary for you to do these calculations using a spreadsheet or a calculator. This procedure, and the statistical tables necessary to decide whether each difference is significant, are covered in more advanced texts such as Zar (1999).

11.6.3 Fixed and random factors

The final complication applies to two factor and more complex analyses of variance that include random factors.

The concept of fixed and random factors was discussed in Section 9.6, but here is a reminder.

A fixed factor is one where the treatments (e.g. levels of temperature) have been **specifically chosen**. You are only interested in those particular treatments and the null hypothesis reflects this – for example, 'There is no difference in cockroach activity at 20°C and 30°C.'

A random factor is one where the treatments are used as random representatives of the full set of possible treatments within that factor. Therefore, the null hypothesis is more general. Instead of comparing specific temperatures the hypothesis is, 'There is no difference in cockroach activity at different temperatures.' The levels of temperature chosen and used in the experiment are merely **random representatives** of the wider range of temperatures that cockroaches may experience.

For a two factor ANOVA both factors could be fixed; one could be random and the other fixed, or both could be random.

Table 11.6. Sources of variation contributing to the mean squares for Factor A, Factor B, and interaction when both A and B are fixed, A is fixed and B is random, and both A and B are random

Source of variation	Both factors fixed	Factor A fixed, B random	Both factors random
Factor A	Factor A + error	Factor A + interaction + error	Factor A + interaction + error
Factor B	Factor B + error	Factor B + error	Factor B + interaction + error
Interaction	Interaction + error	Interaction + error	Interaction + error

If a two factor experiment contains **two fixed factors**, the method for calculating the F ratios for the main effects (Factor A and Factor B) are those given in Table 11.3 and repeated in Table 11.6. The mean square for each factor estimates the effect of that factor plus error, and an F ratio is obtained by dividing the mean square for that factor by the within groups (error) mean square.

If, however, the analysis contains **two random factors**, the sum of squares and mean square for each of the two factors will be **inflated by the inclusion of any additional variation caused by interaction**. Therefore, the variation estimated by the mean square for each main effect will be the effect of that factor, plus interaction plus error. This is explained pictorially below. Most importantly, to realistically estimate the F ratios for each random factor you need to divide the factor mean squares by the interaction MS (which estimates interaction plus error) rather than the error MS (Table 11.6).

Finally, if the ANOVA has **one fixed and one random factor**, it is even more complicated. Most authors recommend that, if Factor A is fixed and Factor B is random, the F ratio for Factor A is obtained by dividing the Factor A MS by the interaction MS, but the F ratio for Factor B is obtained by dividing the Factor B MS by the error MS (Table 11.6). In all cases the F ratio for interaction is obtained by dividing the interaction MS by the error MS.

Importantly, many statistical packages do **not** give appropriate F ratios when random factors are included in an analysis, so you have to do these calculations yourself by dividing by the appropriate mean squares.

Here is a conceptual pictorial explanation for the different ways of estimating main effects in a two factor ANOVA depending on whether the other factor is fixed or random. In all cases the fixed factor of interest is Factor A.

Imagine the hypothetical case where the only levels of Factor A and B that exist in the world are A1 and A2, and B1, B2, B3, and B4. As an example, A1 and A2 may be the only two dietary supplements available for feeding to farmed catfish, of which there are only four species (B1 to B4) and you are interested in the effects of dietary supplements on the growth of these species.

Figure 11.9(a) shows growth for all eight possible combinations of Factors A and B. Note that there is no effect of Factor A when averaged over all possible levels of Factor B, since the means for each of the levels A1 and A2, ignoring the separate levels of Factor B, are the same, but there is considerable interaction between the two factors.

Both factors fixed and an interaction

First, consider the case where **both factors are fixed**, and you are **only interested in the four combinations of A1 and A2 with B2 and B4.** Since both factors are fixed, you are **not** interested in whether any differences in growth between A1 and A2 within this very restricted comparison also reflect those averaged over all possible levels of Factor B.

The comparisons between A1, A2 and B2, B4 are shown in Figure 11.9(b). Cell means have been copied from the appropriate part of Figure 11.9(a). **Although the means of treatments A1 and A2 (ignoring B) are affected by the interaction,** you are only interested in treatment A1 compared with A2 **within the two fixed levels of B2 and B4.** Therefore, to get a realistic effect of Factor A within this limited and fixed comparison, the variation due to the interaction is a necessary additional component of Factor A and you calculate the F ratio for Factor A by dividing its treatment mean square by error only.

Factor A fixed, Factor B random, and an interaction

Second, consider the case where **Factor A is fixed and Factor B is random.** You are interested in the comparison between A1 and A2 across **all possible levels of B**, from which B2 and B4 have been chosen as random representatives.

The results of the experiment on the combinations of A1, A2 and B2, B4 are shown in Figure 11.9(c). Here too, the pooled means of treatments A1 and A2 (ignoring B) are affected by the interaction, but the difference within the experiment **does not reflect the lack of change between A1 and A2 averaged over all possible levels of Factor B in** Figure 11.9(a). Therefore, since the interaction has contributed additional variation to the

(a)

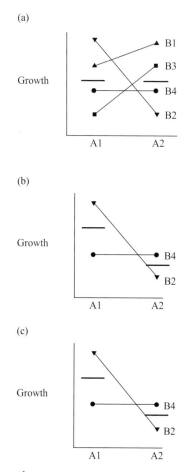

(b)

(c)

Figure 11.9 A pictorial explanation for the reason why the *F* ratio for a main effect is calculated differently, depending on whether the other factor is fixed or random. Cell means are indicated by symbols and pooled treatment means are indicated by the two heavy horizontal lines. (a) All the possible levels of Factor A and Factor B, together with all possible combinations of these, are shown. Note that there is considerable interaction, but overall there is no effect of Factor A (when Factor B is ignored, the pooled treatment means for A1 and A2 are identical). (b) When Factor B is fixed and only a subset of B is considered (B2 and B4), the interaction will contribute to the difference between the pooled means of A1 and A2, but this variation is a relevant addition within the deliberately restricted levels of each factor being compared. (c) When Factor B is random, the interaction will contribute unrealistic additional variation to the difference between the pooled means of A1 and A2. It will not indicate the true lack of change from A1 to A2 across the entire set of the levels of B and therefore needs to be excluded.

sum of squares and mean square for Factor A, it is appropriate to exclude it by dividing the Factor A mean square by the interaction + error mean square to get a more realistic effect of Factor A averaged over all four possible levels of B.

For any two factor ANOVA, the effect of a particular factor (e.g. Factor A) is estimated by dividing by the mean square for error only if the other factor is fixed, but by the mean square for interaction (i.e. interaction + error) if the other factor is random. Therefore, if both factors are random, you divide the mean squares of both by the interaction mean square.

Finally, although I have specified the procedure for obtaining realistic *F* ratios when one or both factors are random, there is still some disagreement about this (e.g. Quinn and Keough, 2002). Some authors recommend dividing the mean square for Factor A and also Factor B by the mean square for interaction + error when either or both are random. Most importantly, if you have an analysis involving one or more random factors, it is important to clearly specify how you calculated the *F* ratios for each factor.

11.7   Unbalanced designs

The cautions about unbalanced designs (when the sample size is not the same in each treatment) in relation to one factor ANOVA also apply to more complex models. Whenever possible you should try to ensure that sample sizes are equal in each treatment combination, especially when sample sizes are relatively small, because they may not give good estimates of cell means and result in misleading conclusions.

11.8   More complex designs

Once you understand the concept of one and two factor analyses of variance, extension to three or more factors and other designs is relatively easy.

A two factor ANOVA breaks the analysis down into two main factors (which are each analysed like a single factor ANOVA) and generates an interaction term by subtraction. A three factor ANOVA does the same thing, but the analysis and ANOVA table are more complex because there are three main factors (Factors A, B, and C), plus interaction among all three ($A \times B$, $A \times C$, $B \times C$, $A \times B \times C$), and error. More advanced texts give rules for obtaining the appropriate *F* ratios with more complex designs, where there can be several combinations of fixed and random factors as well.

If you continue on to use ANOVA a lot, you will realise that this chapter is very introductory. There are nested ANOVAs, two factor ANOVAs without replication, ANOVAs for split plot designs, unbalanced designs, and many more. This book does not attempt to cover all of these – instead it provides you with a general conceptual view that will help you work with more complex designs. Perhaps the best advice if you have to do complex experiments requiring complicated ANOVAs is to find a good textbook (e.g. Quinn and Keough, 2002; Zar, 1999; Sokal and Rohlf, 1995) and perhaps talk to a statistician before you design the experiment.

12 | Important assumptions of analysis of variance: transformations and a test for equality of variances

12.1   Introduction

Parametric analysis of variance assumes the data are from normally distributed populations with the same variance and there is independence, both within and among treatments. If these assumptions are not met, an ANOVA may give you an unrealistic F statistic and therefore an unrealistic probability that several sample means are from the same population. Therefore it is important to know how robust ANOVA is to violations of these assumptions and what to do if they are not met, since in some cases it may be possible to transform the data to make variances more homogeneous or give distributions that are better approximations to the normal curve.

This chapter discusses the assumptions of ANOVA, followed by three frequently used transformations. Finally, there are descriptions of two tests for the homogeneity of variances.

12.2   Homogeneity of variances

The first and most important assumption is that the data for each treatment (or treatment combination in the case of two factor and more complex ANOVA designs) are assumed to have come from populations that have the same variance. Equality of variances is called **homogeneity of variances** or **homoscedasticity**, while unequal variances show **heterogeneity of variances** or **heteroscedasticity**. Nevertheless, statisticians have found that ANOVA is relatively robust in terms of departures from homoscedasticity, and there has been considerable discussion about whether it is necessary to apply tests which assess this before doing an ANOVA, especially since these may be too sensitive when sample sizes are large, or too insensitive when sample sizes are small (e.g. Quinn and Keough, 2002). Many authors suggest preliminary testing for homoscedasticity is **not** necessary, providing as a very general rule the ratio of the difference in variance of the largest to the smallest does not exceed 4:1.

Some cases of heteroscedasticity can be reduced by transforming the data (Section 12.5). Consequently, it is often useful to plot the data or calculate the variance within each treatment, or treatment combination, to see if there is a trend. For example, biological data often show an increase in variance as the mean increases, in which case transforming the data by taking the square root of each value may reduce heteroscedasticity (Section 12.5).

There are several tests designed to assess heteroscedasticity and these have more uses than just checking whether data are suitable for parametric analysis. Sometimes you may be interested in an hypothesis about the **variances** rather than the means of different treatments. For example, you might hypothesise that a drug treatment increases the variance of systolic blood pressure in humans, so you would need to analyse your data with a test that compares variances among treatments. The Levene test for heteroscedasticity is described in Section 12.7.

12.3   Normally distributed data

The second assumption is that the data are from normally distributed populations. Nevertheless, it has been shown that ANOVA is quite robust in terms of minor departures from normality. As previously described in Section 7.7.1, drawing P-P plots can assess normality. You should only be cautious about proceeding with a parametric analysis if a P-P plot shows gross departures from linearity such as sharp kinks.

12.3.1 Skew and outliers

A box and whiskers plot (Tukey, 1977) is a way of visually summarising the distribution of a sample (Figure 12.1) so it can be assessed for **skew** and whether there are values in the data set which are unusually distant (either greater or less) from the mean. These are called **outliers**. Construction of a box and whiskers plot is straightforward.

For a sample containing an odd number of values you need to find the median, which is the middle value of this set of data.

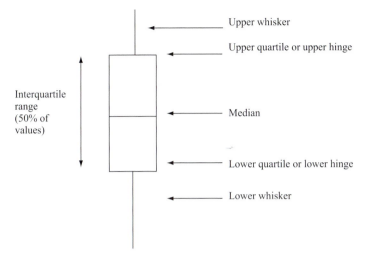

Figure 12.1 The features of a box and whiskers plot.

Next, divide the data into two sets, the first of which contains all the values less than the median and the second of which contains all the values more than the median. Include the median in each set.

Then, find the median of each of the lower and upper set. These new medians are called the **lower quartile** and **upper quartile,** which are used to draw the upper and lower limits (which are also called the **hinges**) of the box. The distance between these quartiles or hinges is the **interquartile range.** Twenty-five per cent of the values in the sample will be larger than the upper quartile, 50% will lie between the two quartiles, and 25% will be smaller than the lower quartile.

Finally, you need to add the whiskers to the box. Each whisker can extend outwards for a maximum distance of 1.5 times the interquartile range from each end of the box, but is only drawn to the **maximum value within that range**.

This will give you a plot with a box running from the lower to upper quartiles and whiskers extending out from each end of the rectangular box (Figure 12.1).

For a data set with an even number of values the procedure is almost the same except that after finding the median you divide the data into two sets, the first of which contains all the values less than the median and the second of which contains all the values more than the median.

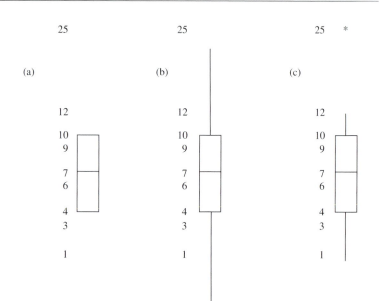

Figure 12.2 The three steps in drawing a box and whiskers plot, using the data in 12.3.2. (a) Drawing the box. (b) Establishing the maximum potential length of each whisker. (c) Drawing the actual length of each whisker.

12.3.2 A worked example of a box and whiskers plot

This example uses a sample with an odd number of values ($n = 9$): 1, 3, 4, 6, 7, 9, 10, 12, 25. The median of this sample is 7, so it is divided into two groups, where the lower group contains 1, 3, 4, 6, and 7, while the upper group contains 7, 9, 10, 12, and 25. The median of the lower group is 4, which becomes the lower quartile. The median of the upper group is 10, which becomes the upper quartile. These are the limits of the ends of the box (called the hinges).

The interquartile range is $10 - 4 = 6$ units. From this you can draw the rectangular box in Figure 12.2(a). The **maximum** potential length of each whisker is 1.5 times the interquartile range and thus $1.5 \times 6 = 9$. This is shown in Figure 12.2(b). Each whisker can extend out a maximum of nine units from its hinge. Since each whisker is only drawn **to the most extreme value within its potential range**, the lower whisker will only extend down to 1, while the upper will only extend up to 12. The outlier of 25, indicated by an asterisk, lies outside the range of the box and its whiskers (Figure 12.2(c)).

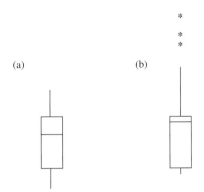

Figure 12.3 Examples of box and whiskers plots for (a) normally distributed data and (b) data with a gross positive skew. Outliers are shown as asterisks.

The **shape** of the box and whiskers plot indicates whether the distribution is skewed. If the distribution of the data is symmetrical about the mean, the box and whiskers plot will have a median equidistant from the hinges and whiskers of similar lengths. As the distribution becomes increasingly skewed, the median will become less equidistant from the hinges and the whiskers will have different lengths (Figure 12.3).

Any values outside the range of the whiskers are called **outliers** and should be scrutinised carefully. In some cases outliers are obvious mistakes caused by incorrect data entry or recording, faulty equipment, or inappropriate methodology (e.g. a human body temperature of 50°C or a negative number of individuals) in which case they can justifiably be deleted. When outliers appear to be real, they are of great interest, since they may indicate that something unusual is occurring, especially if they are present in some samples or treatments and not others. Importantly, however, when there are outliers you should be cautious about using a parametric test. One or two extreme values can greatly affect the variance of a sample, since the formula for the variance uses the square of the difference between each value and the mean, so the assumption of equal variances among treatments or samples can be easily violated.

12.4   Independence

Finally, the data must be independent of each other, both within and among groups. This important assumption needs very little explanation since it is really just a matter of good experimental design. For example, you need to ensure each experimental unit within each treatment is chosen independently and all possible experimental units within the population have an equal likelihood of being selected. You also need to ensure that independence applies among treatment groups as well.

12.5 Transformations

Transformations are a way of reducing heteroscedasticity or making data more closely resemble a normal distribution. There are many transformations available, and three commonly used ones are described below. Most spreadsheet and statistical packages include a large set of transformations.

12.5.1 The square root transformation

If the variance of the data increases as the mean increases, a square root transformation will make these data more homosecdastic. There is an example in Table 12.1.

Table 12.1. An example of the effect of a square root transformation on data where the variance increases as the mean increases. Data are given for the growth of tumours in three drug treatments. The original data show gross heteroscedasticity among groups in that the largest variance is 75.34 and the smallest is 9.00, giving a ratio of largest to smallest of 8.4:1. A square root transformation reduces this ratio to 2.5:1

Control		Tumostat		Inhibin 4	
Original	Square root	Original	Square root	Original	Square root
17	4.12	9	3.00	5	2.24
16	4.00	8	2.83	4	2.00
2	1.41	3	1.73	2	1.41
1	1.00	2	1.41	1	1.00
s^2 75.34	6.92	30.25	5.02	9.00	2.75

(a)

(b)

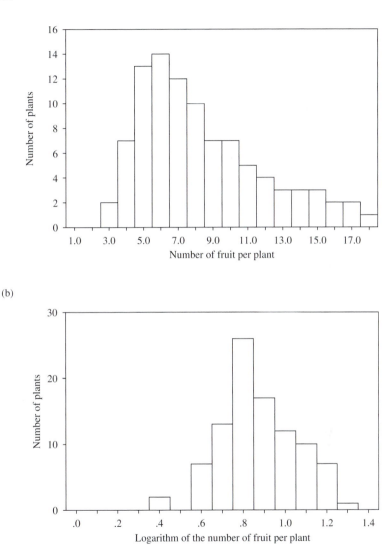

Figure 12.4 The effect of logarithmic transformation on data for the number of fruit produced by tomato plants. The X axis shows the number of fruit produced per plant and the Y axis shows the number of plants bearing each number of fruit. The data show a pronounced positive skew before transformation. (a) Untransformed data show a positive skew. (b) After transformation to the $\log_{10}$. Note that the distribution in (b) is far more symmetrical than in (a).

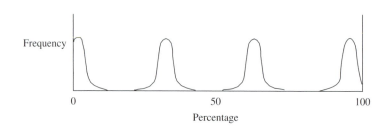

Figure 12.5 Restriction of the normal distribution for percentage data when the mean is close to zero or 100%.

12.5.2 The logarithmic transformation

If the data show a gross positive skew, a logarithmic transformation will give a distribution that better approximates the normal distribution. In cases where the data set includes any values of zero you need to use the logarithm of $X + 1$, since the logarithm of zero is $- \infty$. Biological data often show a positive skew.

Figure 12.4 shows the effect of a logarithmic transformation on a positively skewed distribution.

12.5.3 The arc-sine transformation

The arc-sine transformation can be useful for data that are percentages. Since percentage data have an absolute minimum of 0% and an absolute maximum of 100%, any distribution with a mean close to either of these extremes is unlikely to have a normal distribution because it will cease at these values (Figure 12.5). An arc-sine transformation will give these data a far more normal shape.

12.6   Are transformations legitimate?

Here you may be thinking that transforming data to make them more suitable for parametric statistical analysis sounds like cheating or altering the data to get the result you want.

First, however, transformations are applied to the entire data set, so each value is treated in the same way.

Second, there is no scientific necessity to use the linear base ten scale that we are so familiar with. Many biological relationships between two variables (e.g. the metabolic rate of an invertebrate and temperature, the number of eggs per female toad versus the length of that female) are logarithms, squares, or cubes. The apparently linear pH scale is actually logarithmic – a pH of 4 indicates a ten-fold difference from pH 5 and a 100-fold difference from pH 6. Therefore, in many cases it is actually more appropriate to transform the data so they reflect the underlying relationship.

Importantly, if you transform a set of data, you also need to transform your null and alternate hypotheses. For example, if you were to hypothesise that 'drugs A, B, and C have no effect on the mean blood glucose concentration in humans' but carried out a logarithmic transformation on your data before analysis, your original hypothesis would also have to be transformed to 'drugs A, B, and C have no effect on the mean of the logarithm of blood glucose concentration in humans'.

12.7   Tests for heteroscedasticity

There are several tests designed to examine whether two or more samples appear to have come from populations with the same variance. As mentioned earlier, if you are only interested in whether the data are suitable for a parametric analysis, the general rule that the ratio of the largest variance to the smallest should not exceed 4:1 can be used. If this ratio is greater, it may be useful to examine the data and see where the differences occur, since it may be possible to transform the data so that a parametric analysis can be done.

If, instead, you are interested in testing an hypothesis about the variance of two or more samples, you can use the Levene test, which also gives an F ratio. Remember, however, that a significant result for the Levene test may not mean the data are unsuitable for analysis by ANOVA, which is quite robust to heteroscedasticity.

Levene's original test calculates the **absolute difference** between each replicate and its treatment mean and then does a one factor ANOVA on these differences. The absolute difference is the difference between any two numbers expressed as a positive value. (For example, the difference between 6 and 3 is −3, while the difference between 3 and 6 is +3, but the **absolute difference** in both cases is +3.)

(a)

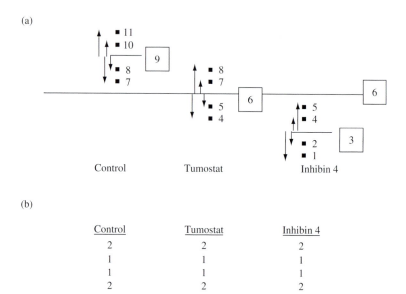

(b)

Control	Tumostat	Inhibin 4
2	2	2
1	1	1
1	1	1
2	2	2

Figure 12.6 The Levene test examines whether two or more variances are likely to have come from the same population by doing a one factor ANOVA on the absolute differences between the replicates and their treatment means or cell means. (a) Arrows show the difference between each replicate and its treatment mean. Note that some differences are positive and some are negative. (b) The absolute differences are listed under each treatment. Every value of the absolute difference between each replicate and its sample mean will be positive. In this case the means of the absolute differences are the same for each treatment, and a one factor ANOVA comparing these will not be significant, thereby indicating the variances are homoscedastic.

Figures 12.6 and 12.7 are a pictorial explanation of the Levene test. Two cases are shown, using the experiment on the growth of brain tumours in three different treatments first described in Section 9.2.

First, if the variances within all treatments are similar, then the set of absolute differences between the replicates and their sample means will also be similar for each treatment. For example, Figure 12.6 shows the absolute differences for three samples that all have the same variance. Note that the means of the absolute differences in 12.6(b) are the same, even though the treatment means in 12.6(a) are not. A one factor ANOVA comparing the means of the absolute differences will not be significant.

(a)

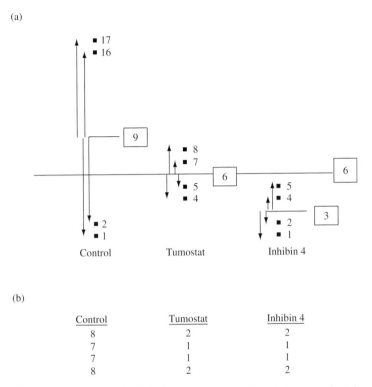

(b)

Control	Tumostat	Inhibin 4
8	2	2
7	1	1
7	1	1
8	2	2

Figure 12.7 An example of the Levene test where there is heteroscedasticity. (a) Arrows show the difference between each replicate and its treatment mean. (b) The absolute differences between each replicate and its treatment mean are listed under each treatment. Since the absolute differences for the control are much greater than the other two treatments a one factor ANOVA comparing the means of the values in (b) will show the variances are significantly heteroscedastic.

Second, if the variances differ among treatments (Figure 12.7(a)), then so will the values of the absolute differences (Figure 12.7(b)). Note that the set of **absolute differences** for the control treatment has a mean that is much larger than the other two and a one factor ANOVA comparing these means is likely to be significant.

The Levene test is available in most statistical packages.

13 | Two factor analysis of variance without replication, and nested analysis of variance

13.1   Introduction

This chapter describes two slightly more complex ANOVA models often used by life scientists, but an understanding of these is **not** essential if you are reading this book as an introduction to biostatistics. If, however, you need to use more complex models, the explanations given here for two factor ANOVA without replication and nested ANOVA are straightforward extensions of the pictorial descriptions in Chapters 9 and 11 and will help with many of the ANOVA models used to analyse more complex designs.

13.2   Two factor ANOVA without replication

This is a special case of the two factor ANOVA described in Chapter 11. Sometimes an orthogonal experiment with two independent factors has to be done without replication, because there is a shortage of experimental subjects or the treatments are very expensive to administer. The simplest case of ANOVA without replication is a two factor design. You cannot do a one factor ANOVA without replication.

The data in Table 13.1 are for a preliminary trial of two experimental drugs 'Proshib' and 'Testoblock', which were being evaluated, together with a control treatment, for their effect on the growth of solid tumours of the prostate, in combination with three levels of radiation therapy (high, medium, and low). The researcher had only nine consenting volunteers with advanced prostate cancer, so an orthogonal design was only possible without replication.

This causes a problem. There is no way to estimate error directly from the dispersion of replicates around their respective cell means (as was done for a one factor ANOVA in Chapter 9 and two factor ANOVA with

Table 13.1. The increase in volume (in mm^3) of prostate tumours in nine males after three months of treatment with nine different combinations of radiation therapy and drugs

Radiation level	Drug		
	Proshib	Testoblock	Control
Low	81	76	79
Medium	45	46	45
High	28	27	27

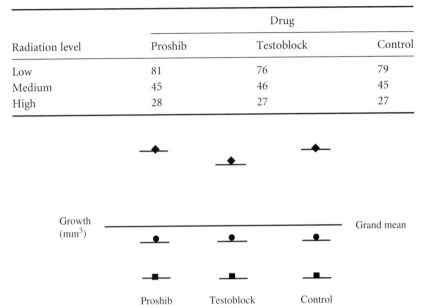

Figure 13.1 The growth of prostate tumours in nine combinations of three levels of drug treatment and three levels of radiation. There is only one replicate within each treatment combination. The increased volume of each tumour is shown as a symbol: ◆ = tumours receiving low radiation, ● = tumours receiving medium radiation, and ■ = tumours receiving high radiation. The heavy horizontal line shows the grand mean and the nine shorter horizontal lines show each cell mean.

replication in Chapter 11), since there is only one value in each treatment combination, so this will be the same as the cell mean. A two factor ANOVA without replication uses a different way of estimating error, which has to assume there is no interaction between the factors.

Figures 13.1 to 13.4 give a pictorial explanation of how a two factor ANOVA without replication estimates three sources of variation and uses these to isolate the effects of the two factors. The data in Table 13.1 are graphed in Figure 13.1.

First, the total variation within the experiment is estimated. Each point will be displaced from the grand mean by the effects of Factor A, Factor B,

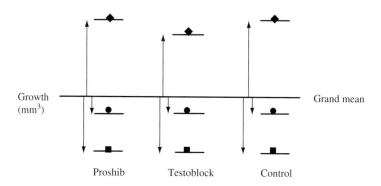

Figure 13.2 The total variation within the experiment on the growth of prostate tumours. The heavy horizontal line indicates the grand mean and the nine shorter horizontal lines indicate each cell mean. The displacement of each point from the grand mean (arrows) will be caused by the total variation within the experiment.

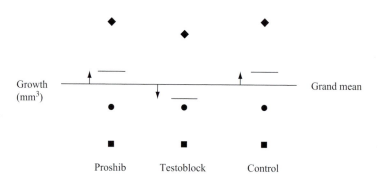

Figure 13.3 Estimation of the effect of Factor A. The displacement of each treatment mean from the grand mean (arrows) will be caused by the effect of Factor A (here drugs) plus error.

any interaction, and error. These distances can be squared and summed to give the sum of squares for the total variation in the experiment, with degrees of freedom that are one less than the number of experimental subjects.

Second, the effect of Factor A is estimated by ignoring Factor B and calculating a new mean for each of the levels within Factor A. The displacement of each treatment mean from the grand mean will be caused by the average effect of Factor A plus error (Figure 13.3). Each of these is squared, multiplied by the number of replicates within each treatment, and added

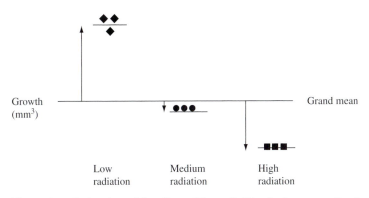

Figure 13.4 Estimation of the effect of Factor B. The displacement of each treatment mean from the grand mean (arrows) will be caused by the effect of Factor B (here radiation) plus error.

together to give the sum of squares for Factor A. The number of degrees of freedom is one less than the number of treatments, and dividing the sum of squares by this value will give the mean square for Factor A.

Finally, the effect of Factor B is estimated by ignoring Factor A and calculating a new mean for each treatment level of Factor B. The displacement of each treatment mean from the grand mean will be caused by the effect of Factor B plus error (Figure 13.4). Here too, the displacements are squared, multiplied by the number of replicates within each treatment, and added together to give the sum of squares for Factor B. The number of degrees of freedom is one less than the number of treatments, and dividing by this value will give the mean square for Factor B.

At this stage you have estimates for the following sources of variation:

(a) **The total variation in the experiment** (the combined effects of Factor A, Factor B, A × B, and error) (Figure 13.2).
(b) **The effect of Factor A** (drug treatment + error) (Figure 13.3).
(c) **The effect of Factor B** (radiation level + error) (Figure 13.4).

Since there is only one replicate within each treatment combination, there is no way to separately estimate error. Therefore, unlike a two factor ANOVA with replication, it is not possible to estimate the sum of squares for the effect of any interaction by subtracting the sums of squares for Factor A, Factor B, and error from the total variation.

Two factor ANOVA without replication does the next best thing. The sums of squares and degrees of freedom in an ANOVA are **additive**

Table 13.2. Results of a two factor ANOVA without replication on the data in Table 13.1. There is a significant effect of radiation but no significant effect of the drugs on the growth of tumours of the prostate

Source of variation	Sum of squares	df	Mean square	F	P
Radiation	4070.222	2	2035.111	835.545	0.000
Drug	4.222	2	2.111	0.864	0.488
Error	9.778	4	2.444		
Total	4084.222	8			

(e.g. in Chapter 9 it was explained how the total sum of squares and total degrees of freedom in a one factor ANOVA were the sums of those for Factor A and for error). Therefore, by subtracting the sums of squares for Factor A plus Factor B from the total variation, you are left with the sum of squares for the remaining variation in the experiment, which will include error and any effect of interaction. This sum of squares, which is the only possible estimate of error, is divided by the remaining degrees of freedom to give the best estimate of the mean square for error. If there is an interaction, the mean square will be inflated, but this is unavoidable and undetectable if you do a two factor ANOVA without replication.

The results of a two factor ANOVA without replication will include the sums of squares and mean squares for Factor A, Factor B, and error, together with the F ratios and probabilities for Factors A and B. For the example given above the results of the analysis are in Table 13.2.

13.3   A-posteriori comparison of means after a two factor ANOVA without replication

If a two factor ANOVA without replication shows a significant effect of a fixed treatment factor (e.g. the three radiation levels being specifically compared in Section 13.2), you are likely to want to know which treatments appear to be from the same or different populations.

The procedure for a-posteriori testing is a modification of the formula for a one factor ANOVA, except that, since there is no directly estimated value for error, the MS error for interaction plus error (estimated by subtraction) is used as the best estimate of this. For a Tukey test each factor is examined separately using the formula:

$$q = \frac{\bar{X}_A - \bar{X}_B}{\text{SEM}} \qquad (13.1) \text{ copied from } (10.1)$$

with the standard error of the mean estimated from:

$$\text{SEM} = \sqrt{\frac{\text{MS error}}{n}} \qquad (13.2) \text{ copied from } (10.3)$$

where the MS error is also the one calculated by subtraction in the ANOVA table (see Table 13.2) and n is the number of data within each group (for example, there are three values within each of the three radiation levels when the drug treatments are ignored and *vice versa*).

13.4 Randomised blocks

Two factor ANOVA without replication can be used to analyse results from a **randomised block** experimental design. Many agricultural experiments on the productivity of commercial crops are done on a large scale and involve treatments applied to particular plots within a field or paddock. When each plot is harvested, you usually only get one value (e.g. the weight of the crop harvested from that plot).

Unfortunately, factors including soil fertility, wind exposure, and soil type may vary across fields and paddocks. Therefore, if you use an experimental design with several replicates of each treatment allocated at random, you may get a lot of variation among replicates of the same treatment simply due to their different locations.

A randomised block design gives a way of isolating treatment effects from this type of spatial variation. An area of land is subdivided into several rows (which are called blocks). Each block is then subdivided into several plots of equal size, usually with one plot for each treatment type. One replicate of each treatment is assigned at random within each block, as shown in Figure 13.5.

The results from this design can be analysed as a two factor ANOVA without replication, using treatments as the first factor and blocks as the second.

Two factor ANOVA without replication is often used to analyse experiments on animals, where you might expect great variation among the offspring of different parents. For example, small mammals usually only have relatively few individuals per litter (e.g. cats have an average of about

Block number				
1	A	C	B	D
2	D	A	B	C
3	C	B	D	A
4	A	D	C	B
5	B	C	D	A

Figure 13.5 An example of a randomised block experimental design. The grid represents a paddock that has been subdivided into several rows, which are treated as separate blocks. Each block has been subdivided into four equal-sized plots. One replicate of each treatment (A–D) is assigned at random to a plot within each block.

three kittens per litter) and there is likely to be considerable genetic variation among litters from different females. In such cases the best approach is often to treat litters as one (random) factor and your treatments as the second factor, with each treatment applied to one individual per litter. Here the factor 'litters' is equivalent to the blocks in the previous example.

13.5   Nested ANOVA as a special case of a one factor ANOVA

An experimental design that compares the means of two or more levels of the same factor (e.g. different levels of salinity or different drugs) can be analysed by a single factor ANOVA, as described in Chapter 9. Sometimes, however, researchers do an experiment with two or more levels of a particular factor, but also have **two or more subgroups nested within each level**. Here is an example.

Large-scale experiments in aquaculture are often constrained by the number of ponds available to the researcher. For example, only nine ponds were available for an investigation into the effects of two different vitamin supplements (vitamin A and vitamin B) on the growth of prawns. Each pond was stocked with 100 prawns of the same species, age, and weight. Three ponds were allocated at random to each of the two vitamin supplement treatments

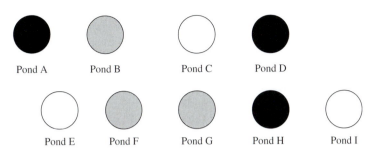

Figure 13.6 Example of a nested or hierarchical design. Each pond contains 100 replicates and three ponds are nested within each treatment. Open circles indicate the control (prawn food only), grey circles treatment 1 (prawn food plus vitamin A), and black circles treatment 2 (prawn food plus vitamin B).

and the remaining three ponds used as a control. After six months the 100 prawns in each pond were recaptured and weighed.

This is called a **nested** or **hierarchical** design. Three ponds, each containing several replicates (in this case 100), are nested within each treatment (Figure 13.6).

This design is not appropriate for analysis using a one factor ANOVA with diet as the factor and the 300 prawns within each treatment as the number of replicates, since this ignores the presence of the ponds that may contribute to the variation within the experiment. You may also be thinking that the design appears pseudoreplicated in that the real level of replication within each treatment is the number of ponds rather than the number of prawns. This is true and the nested analysis described below takes this into account.

This design is also unsuitable for analysis as a two factor ANOVA with diet as the first factor and ponds as the second, because the three ponds are simply random subgroups nested within each treatment, which do not intentionally contain different levels of a second factor. For example, the first pond in treatment 1 does not share an exclusive property with the first pond in treatments 2 and 3 (Table 13.3).

When one factor (e.g. Factor B) is nested within another (e.g. Factor A) it is often written as Factor B(Factor A). For the nested design above, where Factor A is diet and Factor B is the ponds, the following will contribute to the final weight of each prawn:

$$\text{Growth} = \text{Factor A} + \text{Factor B(FactorA)} + \text{error} \tag{13.3}$$

Table 13.3. A hierarchical design should not be analysed as an independent factor design

(a) A hierarchical design has one factor nested within the other. The ponds have been chosen at random and are nested within each treatment.

	Prawn food			Prawn food + vitamin A			Prawn food + vitamin B		
Pond C	Pond E	Pond I	Pond B	Pond F	Pond G	Pond A	Pond D	Pond H

(b) Incorrect format of the nested design shown above in (a) as a fully orthogonal design. There is nothing exclusively shared within any of the rows of ponds across treatments so it is incorrect to treat the three rows as three different levels of the factor 'pond'.

	Treatment		
Pond	Prawn food	Prawn food + vitamin A	Prawn food + vitamin B
First within each treatment	100 prawns (Pond C)	100 prawns (Pond B)	100 prawns (Pond A)
Second within each treatment	100 prawns (Pond E)	100 prawns (Pond F)	100 prawns (Pond D)
Third within each treatment	100 prawns (Pond I)	100 prawns (Pond G)	100 prawns (Pond H)

This is the same as equation (9.1) for a one factor ANOVA apart from an additional source of variation from the ponds nested within each diet. There is no interaction term because the design is not orthogonal.

A nested ANOVA isolates the effects of treatments and subgroups within these treatments and gives an F ratio for both factors. The way this analysis works is described in Section 13.6.

13.6   A pictorial explanation of a nested ANOVA

For simplicity the following example has two treatments and two ponds nested within each treatment, with only four prawns in each pond. The data are in Table 13.4. Diet is Factor A and the ponds are Factor B(A).

Table 13.4. Data for the weight in grams of prawns after six weeks of feeding with (a) standard prawn food plus vitamin A and (b) standard prawn food only. Two ponds are nested within each treatment

Treatment			
Prawn food + vitamin A		Prawn food only	
Pond 1	Pond 2	Pond 3	Pond 4
30	60	80	110
35	65	85	115
45	75	95	125
50	80	100	130

Figure 13.7 shows the data for each of the four groups in Table 13.4 graphed as four separate cells, including each cell mean and the grand mean.

First, error is estimated. The value for each replicate is displaced from its cell mean by error only (Figure 13.7). The sum of squares for error is obtained by squaring each displacement and adding these together. This quantity is divided by the appropriate degrees of freedom (the sum of one less than the number of replicates within each of the cells) to give the mean square for error.

Second, the subgroups (in this case the ponds) are ignored and new means are calculated by combining all of the replicates within each treatment (in this case diet) (Figure 13.8). This will give the effect of treatment, but for a nested ANOVA each treatment mean will be displaced from the grand mean because of the **effect of treatment, plus the subgroups nested within each treatment, plus error**.

This seems inconsistent with the explanation given for an orthogonal two factor ANOVA, where ignoring a factor (e.g. Factor B) removed it as a source of variation, allowing the effect of the other (e.g. Factor A) to be estimated. For a two factor orthogonal design, all levels of Factor A are present within every level of Factor B and vice versa, so each of the two factors can be ignored in turn and the effect of each factor separately estimated. For a nested design, however, the effects of Factor B (the subgroups) cannot be excluded in this way, because **different** subgroups (here different ponds) are present and may contribute very different amounts of variation within each of the levels of Factor A.

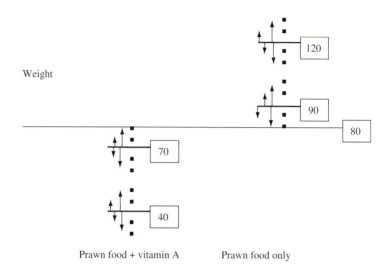

Figure 13.7 Arrows show the displacement of each replicate from its cell mean, which is the variation due to error only. The number of degrees of freedom is the sum of one less than the number within each of the cells. In this example there are 12 degrees of freedom.

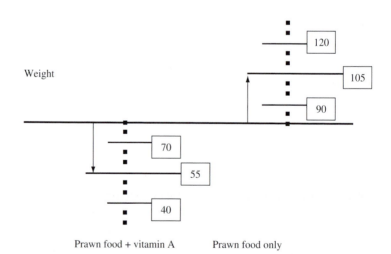

Figure 13.8 Estimation of the effects of Factor A (treatment). The displacement of each combined treatment mean for Factor A from the grand mean shown by the arrows is caused by the average effects of that treatment, plus ponds nested within each treatment, plus error. The number of degrees of freedom will be one less than the number of treatments, so in this example with two treatments there is one degree of freedom.

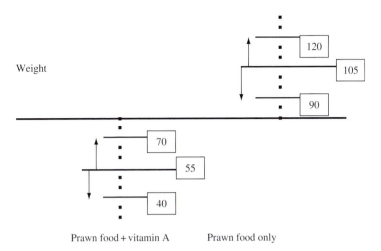

Figure 13.9 Estimation of the effect of Factor B(A). The displacement of each cell mean from its treatment mean is shown by each arrow and is caused by the average effect of that subgroup (each pond) plus error. The number of degrees of freedom will be the sum of one less than the number of ponds within each treatment. In this example there are two degrees of freedom.

The displacements of each treatment mean from the grand mean are squared, multiplied by the number of replicates within their respective treatment, and added together to give the sum of squares for Factor A, which will include treatment, plus subgroups(treatment), plus error. The number of degrees of freedom is one less than the number of treatments, and dividing the sum of squares by this number will give the mean square for Factor A (i.e. treatment plus subgroups(treatment), plus error).

Third, a mean is also calculated for Factor B(A), which is the variation contributed by each subgroup (in this case each pond) (Figure 13.9). Each subgroup mean will only be displaced from its respective treatment mean by the effect of the subgroup plus error. The displacements are squared, multiplied by the number of replicates within their respective subgroups and added together to give the Factor B(A) sum of squares. The number of degrees of freedom will be the sum of one less than the number of subgroups within each treatment. Dividing the sum of squares by this number will give the mean square for Factor B(A) (i.e. subgroups plus error).

Table 13.5. The appropriate division and components of each mean square term used to estimate the effect of each factor when Factor B is nested within Factor A

Source of variation	Calculation of F ratio	Components of each mean square
Factor A (treatment)		
	$\dfrac{\text{Mean square for Factor A}}{\text{Mean square for B(A)}}$	$\dfrac{\text{Factor A + Factor B(A) + error}}{\text{Factor B(A) + error}}$
Factor B(A) (subgroups nested within each treatment)	$\dfrac{\text{Mean square for B(A)}}{\text{Mean square error}}$	$\dfrac{\text{Factor B(A) + error}}{\text{error}}$

The procedures shown in Figures 13.7 to 13.9 give three separate sums of squares and mean squares:

(a) Factor A: treatment + subgroups(treatment) + error (Figure 13.8)
(b) Factor B(A): subgroups(treatment) + error (Figure 13.9)
(c) error (Figure 13.7)

and no other mean squares are needed to isolate the effects of the treatments from the subgroups nested within each treatment.

First, to isolate the effect of treatment only, the MS for treatment plus subgroups(treatment) plus error is divided by the MS for subgroups(treatment) plus error. Second, to isolate the variation due to subgroups(treatment), the MS for subgroups(treatment) plus error is divided by the MS error (Table 13.5).

In the example shown in Figures 13.7 to 13.9 the F ratio for the effect of Factor A will only have one and two degrees of freedom, despite there being 16 prawns in the experiment. This is appropriate because the level of replication for this comparison is the ponds rather than the prawns within each pond.

Most statistical packages will do a nested ANOVA and the results will be in a similar format to Table 13.6, which gives the results for the data in Table 13.4. If the treatment factor is fixed and significant, you are likely to want to carry out a-posteriori testing to examine which treatment means are

Table 13.6. Results of a nested ANOVA on the data in Table 13.4. Note that the *F* ratio for diet has been obtained by dividing the MS for diet by the MS for pond (diet)

Source of variation	Sum of squares	df	Mean square	*F*	*P*
Diet	10000.0	1	10000.0	5.556	0.143
Pond(diet)	3600.0	2	1800.0	21.600	0.000
Error	1000.0	12	83.3		

significantly different. The Tukey test (equation (13.1)) can be used, but when comparing among treatments the appropriate 'MS error' to use in equation (13.3) is the MS for subgroups(treatments) instead of the error. I suggest you use a more advanced text (e.g. Sokal and Rohlf (1995) or Zar (1999)) if you need to do a-posteriori testing after a nested ANOVA.

This example is the simplest case of a nested or hierarchical design. More complex designs can include several levels of nesting, and nested factors in combination with two and higher factor ANOVAs. If you need to use more complex designs, it is important to read an advanced text or talk to a statistician before doing the experiment.

13.7   A final comment on ANOVA – this book is only an introduction

Even though this book has five chapters about analysis of variance, it is only an introduction to an enormous and diverse topic. There are far more complex ANOVA models, including those for analysing repeated measures on the same experimental unit over time, several variables measured on the same experimental unit, and designs with several factors that include nesting. Hopefully the introduction developed here will make it easier for you to understand more complex designs described in advanced texts!

14 | Relationships between variables: linear correlation and linear regression

14.1   Introduction

Often life scientists obtain data for two or more variables measured on the same set of subjects or experimental units because they are interested in whether these variables are **related** and, if so, the **type of functional relationship** between them.

If two variables are related they **vary together** – as the value of one variable increases or decreases, the other also changes in a consistent way.

If two variables are **functionally related,** they vary together and the value of one variable can be predicted from the value of the other.

To detect a relationship between two variables, both are measured on each of several subjects or experimental units and these **bivariate data** examined to see if there is any pattern. One way to do this, by drawing a scatter plot with one variable on the X axis and the other on the Y axis, was described in Chapter 3, but, although this can reveal patterns, it does not show whether two variables are **significantly related**, or have a **significant functional relationship**. This is another case where you have to use a statistical test, because an apparent relationship between two variables may only have occurred by chance in a sample from a population where there is no relationship. A statistic will indicate the strength of the relationship, together with the probability of getting that particular result, or an outcome even more extreme, in a sample from a population where there is **no relationship** between the two variables.

Two parametric methods for statistically analysing relationships between variables are **linear correlation** and **linear regression**, both of which can be used on data measured on a ratio, interval, or ordinal scale. Correlation and regression have very different uses, and there have been many cases where correlation has been inappropriately used instead of regression and *vice versa.* After contrasting correlation and regression, this chapter explains correlation analysis. Regression analysis is explained in Chapter 15.

14.2   Correlation contrasted with regression

Correlation is an **exploratory** technique used to examine whether the values of two variables are significantly **related,** meaning whether the values of both variables change together in a consistent way. (For example, an increase in one may be accompanied by a decrease in the other.) **There is no expectation that the value of one variable can be predicted from the other, or that there is any causal relationship between them.**

In contrast, regression analysis is used to **describe the functional relationship** between two variables so that the value of one can be predicted from the other. A functional relationship means that the value of one variable (called the **dependent** variable) can **be determined** by the value of the second (the **independent** variable), but the reverse is not true. For example, the amount of tooth wear in koala bears, which feed on leaves, is likely to be determined by age, because older koalas will have spent more time chewing. The opposite is not true – the age of a koala bear is not determined by how worn its teeth are! Nevertheless, although tooth wear is determined by age, it is not **caused** by age – it is actually caused by chewing. This is an important point. Regression analysis can be used provided there is a good reason to hypothesise that one variable (the dependent one) can be determined by another (the independent one), but it does not necessarily have to be caused by it.

Regression analysis provides an equation that describes the **functional relationship** between two variables and which can be used to predict values of the dependent variable from the independent one. The very different uses of correlation and regression are summarised in Table 14.1.

14.3   Linear correlation

The Pearson correlation coefficient, symbolised by ρ (the Greek letter rho) for a population and by r for a sample, is a statistic that indicates the extent to which two variables are linearly related, and can be any value from -1 to $+1$. Usually the population statistic ρ is not known, so it is estimated by the sample statistic r.

Table 14.1. A contrast between the uses of correlation and regression

Correlation	Regression
Exploratory – are two variables significantly related?	Definitive – what is the functional relationship between variable Y and variable X and is it significant? Predictive – what is the value of Y given a particular value of X?
Neither Y nor X has to be dependent upon the other variable. Neither variable has to be determined by the other.	Variable Y is dependent upon X, but the reverse is not true. It must be plausible that Y is determined by X, but Y does not necessarily have to be caused by X.

An r of $+1$, which shows a perfect positive linear correlation, will only be obtained when the values of both variables increase together and lie along a straight line (Figure 14.1(a)). Similarly, an r of -1, which shows a perfect negative linear correlation, will only be obtained when the value of one variable decreases as the other increases and the points also lie along a straight line (Figure 14.1(b)). In contrast, an r of zero shows the lack of a relationship between two variables and Figure 14.1(c) gives one example where the points lie along a straight line parallel to the X axis. When the points are more scattered but both variables tend to increase together, the values of r will be between zero and $+1$ (Figure 14.1(d)), while, if one variable tends to decrease as the other increases, the value of r will be between zero and -1 (Figure 14.1(e)). If there is no relationship and considerable scatter (Figure 14.1(f)), the value of r will be close to zero. Finally, it is important to remember that linear correlation will only detect a linear relationship between variables – even though the two variables shown in Figure 14.1(g) are obviously related the value of r will be close to zero.

14.4   Calculation of the Pearson r statistic

A statistic for correlation needs to reliably describe the strength of a linear relationship for any bivariate data set, even when the two variables have

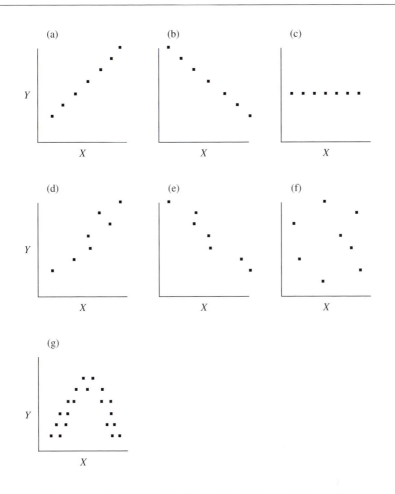

Figure 14.1 Some examples of the value of the correlation coefficient *r*.
(a) A perfect linear relationship where $r = 1$. (b) A perfect linear relationship
where $r = -1$. (c) No relationship ($r = 0$). (d) A positive linear relationship
with $0 < r < 1$. (e) A negative linear relationship where $-1 < r < 0$. (f) No
linear relationship (*r* is close to zero). (g) An obvious relationship, but one
that will not be detected by linear correlation (*r* will be close to zero).

been measured on very different scales. For example, the values of one
variable might range from zero to 10, while the other might range from zero
to 1000. To obtain a statistic that always has a value between 1 and −1, with
these maximum and minimum values indicating a perfect positive and
negative linear relationship respectively, you need a way of standardising

the data. This is straightforward and is done by transforming the values of both variables to Z scores, as described in Chapter 6.

To transform a set of data to Z scores, the mean is subtracted from each value and the result divided by the standard deviation. This will give a distribution that **always** has a mean of zero and a standard deviation (and variance) of 1. For a population the equation for Z is:

$$Z = \frac{X_i - \mu}{\sigma} \qquad \text{(14.1) copied from (6.3)}$$

and for a sample it is:

$$Z = \frac{X_i - \bar{X}}{s} \qquad (14.2)$$

Figure 14.2 shows the effect of transforming bivariate data measured on different scales to their Z scores.

Once the data for both variables have been converted to their Z scores it is easy to calculate a statistic that indicates the strength of the relationship between them.

If the two increase together, large positive values of Z_x will always be associated with large positive values of Z_y and large negative values of Z_x will also be associated with large negative values of Z_y (Figure 14.3(a)).

If there is no relationship between the variables, all of the values of Z_y will be zero (Figure 14.3(b)).

Finally, if one variable decreases as the other increases, large positive values of Z_x will be consistently associated with large negative values of Z_y and *vice versa* (Figure 14.3(c)).

This gives a way of calculating a comparative statistic that indicates the extent to which the two variables are related. If the Z_x and Z_y scores for each of the experimental units are multiplied together and summed (equation (14.3)), data with a positive correlation will give a total with a positive value, while data with a negative correlation will give a total with a negative one. In contrast, data for two variables that are not related will give a total close to zero:

$$\sum_{i=1}^{n} (Z_{xi} \times Z_{yi}) \qquad (14.3)$$

Importantly, the largest possible positive value of $\sum_{i=1}^{n} (Z_{xi} \times Z_{yi})$ will be obtained when each pair of data has exactly the same Z scores for both

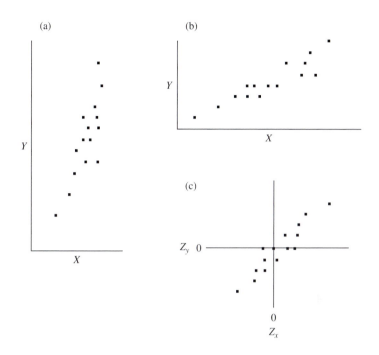

Figure 14.2 For any set of data, dividing the distance between each value and the mean by the standard deviation will give a mean of zero and a standard deviation (and variance) of 1.0. The scales on which X and Y have been measured are very different for cases (a) and (b) above, but transformation of both variables gives the distribution shown in (c), where both Z_x and Z_y have a mean of zero and a standard deviation of 1.0.

variables (Figure 14.3(a)) and the largest possible negative value will be obtained when the Z scores for each pair of data are the same number but opposite in sign (Figure 14.3(c)). If the pairs of scores do not vary together completely in either a positive or negative way, the total will be a smaller positive (Figure 14.3(d)) or negative number (Figure 14.3(f)).

This total will increase as the size of the sample increases, so dividing by the degrees of freedom (N for a population and $n-1$ for a sample) will give a statistic that has been 'averaged', just as the equation for the standard deviation and variance of a sample are averaged and corrected for sample size by dividing by $n-1$. The statistic given by equation (14.4) is the Pearson correlation coefficient r.

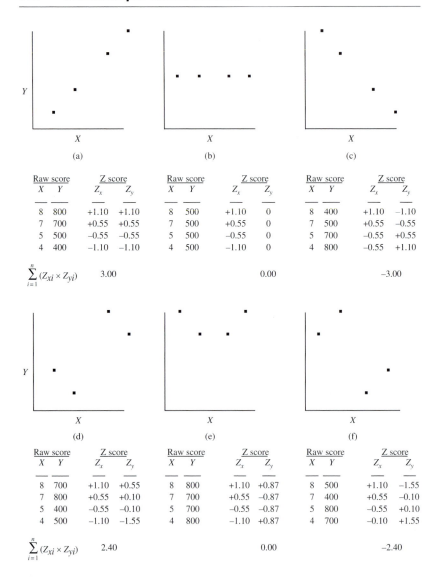

Figure 14.3 Examples of raw scores and Z scores for data with (a) a perfect positive linear relationship (all points lie along a straight line), (b) no relationship, (c) a perfect negative linear relationship (all points lie along a straight line), (d) a positive relationship, (e) no relationship, and (f) a negative relationship. Note that the largest positive and negative values for the sum of the products of the two Z scores for each point occur when there is a perfect positive or negative relationship, and that these values ($+3$ and -3) are equivalent to $n-1$ and $-(n-1)$ respectively.

$$r = \frac{\sum\limits_{i=1}^{n} (Z_{xi} \times Z_{yi})}{n - 1} \tag{14.4}$$

More importantly, equation (14.4) gives a statistic that will only ever be between -1 and $+1$. This is easy to show. In Chapter 6 it was described how the Z distribution always has a mean of zero and a standard deviation (and variance) of 1.0. If you were to calculate the variance of the Z scores for only one variable, you would use the equation:

$$s^2 = \frac{\sum\limits_{i=1}^{n} (Z_i - \bar{Z})^2}{n - 1} \tag{14.5}$$

but, since $\bar{Z}$ is zero, this equation becomes:

$$s^2 = \frac{\sum\limits_{i=1}^{n} Z_i^2}{n - 1} \tag{14.6}$$

and, since s^2 is always 1 for the Z distribution, the numerator of equation (14.6) is always equal to $n - 1$.

Therefore, for a set of bivariate data where the two Z scores within each experimental unit are **exactly the same in magnitude and sign**, the equation for the correlation between the two variables:

$$r = \frac{\sum\limits_{i=1}^{n} (Z_{xi} \times Z_{yi})}{n - 1} \tag{14.7}$$

will be equivalent to:

$$r = \frac{\sum\limits_{i=1}^{n} Z_{xi}^2}{n - 1} \quad \text{or} \quad \frac{n - 1}{n - 1} = 1.0 \tag{14.8}$$

Consequently, when there is perfect agreement between Z_x and Z_y for each point, the value of r will be 1.0. If the Z scores generally increase together but not all the points lie along a straight line, the value of r will be between zero and 1 because the numerator of equation (14.8) will be less than $n - 1$.

Similarly, if every Z score for the first variable is the **exact negative equivalent** of the other, the numerator of equation (14.8) will be the negative equivalent of $n-1$ so the value of r will be -1.0. If one variable decreases while the other increases but not all the points lie along a straight line, the value of r will be between -1.0 and zero.

Finally, for a set of points along any line parallel to the X axis, all of the Z scores for the Y variable will be zero, so the value of the numerator of equation (14.6) and r will also be zero.

14.5   Is the value of *r* statistically significant?

Having obtained the value of r, you need to establish whether it is significantly different to zero. Statisticians have calculated the distribution of r for random samples of different sizes taken from a population where there is no correlation between two variables. When $\rho = 0$, the distribution of values of r for many samples taken from that population will be normally distributed with a mean of zero. Both positive and negative values of r will be generated by chance, and 5% of these will be greater than a positive critical value or less than its negative equivalent. The critical value will depend on the size of the sample, and as sample size increases the value of r is likely to become closer to the value of ρ. Statistical packages will calculate r and give the probability the sample has been taken from a population where $\rho = 0$.

14.6   Assumptions of linear correlation

Linear correlation analysis assumes that the data are random representatives taken from the larger population of values for each variable, which are normally distributed and have been measured on a ratio, interval or ordinal scale. A scatter plot of these variables will have what is called a **bivariate normal distribution**. If the data are not normally distributed, or the relationship does not appear to be linear, they may be able to be analysed by nonparametric tests for correlation, which are described in Chapter 17.

14.7   Summary and conclusion

Correlation is an exploratory technique used to test whether two variables are related. It is often useful to draw a scatter plot of the data to see if there is any pattern before calculating the correlation coefficient, since the variables may be related together in a non-linear way. The Pearson correlation coefficient is a statistic that shows the extent to which two variables are linearly related, and can have a value between -1.0 and 1.0, with these extremes showing a perfect negative linear relationship and perfect positive linear relationship respectively, while zero shows no relationship. The value of r indicates the way in which the variables are related, but the probability of getting a particular r value is needed to decide whether the correlation is statistically significant.

15 | Simple linear regression

15.1 Introduction

This chapter explains how simple linear regression analysis describes the functional relationship between a dependent and an independent variable. The different uses of correlation and regression were contrasted in Chapter 14. Correlation examines if two variables are related. Regression describes the **functional relationship** between a dependent and an independent variable.

15.2 Linear regression

Linear regression analysis is often used by life scientists. For example, the equation for the regression of one variable on another may suggest hypotheses about why the two variables are functionally related. More practically, regression can be used in situations where the dependent variable is difficult, expensive or impossible to measure, but its values can be predicted from another easily measured variable to which it is functionally related. Here is an example.

There is considerable variation in the height of adult humans. Consequently, parents who have a child that is relatively short for its age often become concerned that it will be relatively short when it becomes an adult. It is easy to make a person grow taller by administering human growth hormone, but this treatment becomes less and less effective after the age of ten and ineffective after about the age of 17. It also has to be used with caution because only small amounts of hormone can cause a considerable increase in growth. Nevertheless, it has been shown that the amount of extra height by which a person will grow can be predicted from the length of uncalcified cartilaginous bone remaining

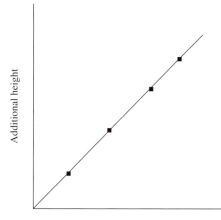

Length of uncalcified bone at age six

Figure 15.1 An example of the use of regression. The additional height by which a child will grow (the dependent variable) can be accurately predicted from the length of uncalcified bone remaining in the fingers at the age of six years (the independent variable). The additional height is determined by and easy to predict from the independent variable, but is not caused by it.

in the bones of their fingers, which can be accurately measured from an x-ray of their hands at quite a young age (e.g. six years). Additional growth is therefore dependent upon (but not caused by) the length of uncalcified bone remaining in the fingers and can be predicted from it by using a regression line (Figure 15.1). If the predicted height is considered unacceptably short by the parents, they may ask for their child to be given additional growth hormone. This is another deliberate example where the dependent variable is not caused by the independent variable but is plausibly determined by it.

A linear regression analysis gives an equation for a line that describes the functional relationship between two variables and tests whether the statistics that describe this line are significantly different to zero.

The simplest functional relationship between a dependent and independent variable is a straight line. Only two statistics, the intercept a (which is the value of Y when X is zero) and the slope of the line b, are needed to uniquely describe where that line occurs on a graph.

The position of any point on a straight line can be described by the equation:

$$Y = a + bX \qquad (15.1)$$

where 'a' is the value of Y when $X = 0$, and b is the slope of the line. For example, the equation $Y = 6 + 0.5X$ means, 'The Y value is 6 units plus half the value of X.' Therefore, for this line, when $X = 0$, $Y = 6$, and, when $X = 10$, $Y = 11$.

Simple linear regression analysis gives an equation for a straight line that is the 'best fit' through a set of data points. It is very easy to obtain a and b if all the points lie on a straight line. When the points are scattered, which they usually are for biological data, the method for obtaining these statistics is also straightforward.

15.3   Calculation of the slope of the regression line

The slope of the regression line is the amount by which the value of Y increases in relation to an increase in the value of X. For example, if an increase in the value of X by one unit is also accompanied by a one unit increase in the value of Y, the slope of the line is 1.0. If, however, the value of Y decreases by three units for every one unit increase in X, then the slope is -3.0.

If all points lie along a straight line, you can calculate the slope by taking any two points and using the equation:

$$b = \frac{Y_2 - Y_1}{X_2 - X_1} \qquad (15.2)$$

which divides the relative change in Y by the relative change in X (Figure 15.2).

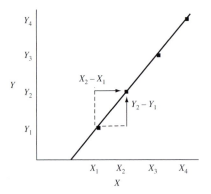

Figure 15.2 Calculation of the slope when all points lie along a straight line. The vertical arrow shows the relative change in Y from Y_1 to Y_2 that occurs with an increase in X from X_1 to X_2 shown by the horizontal arrow. For any two points, $Y_2 - Y_1$ divided by $X_2 - X_1$ will give the slope, which in this case is positive since Y increases as X increases and vice versa.

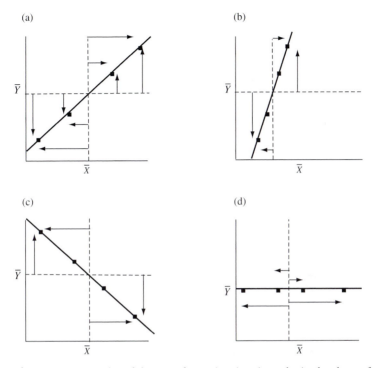

Figure 15.3 Examples of the use of equation (15.3) to obtain the slope of the regression line. Vertical arrows show $Y_i - \bar{Y}$ and horizontal arrows show $X_i - \bar{X}$. (a) For every point along a line with a slope of 1.0, $Y_i - \bar{Y}$ will be the same magnitude and sign as $X_i - \bar{X}$, so equation (15.3) will give a value of 1.0. (b) For every point along a line with a slope of 3.0, $Y_i - \bar{Y}$ will be the same sign but three times greater than $X_i - \bar{X}$, so equation (15.3) will give a value of 3.0. (c) For every point along a line with a slope of -1.0, $Y_i - \bar{Y}$ will be the same magnitude but opposite sign as $X_i - \bar{X}$, so equation (15.3) will give a value of -1.0. (d) For a slope of zero, each value of $Y_i - \bar{Y}$ will be zero, so equation (15.3) will give a value of zero.

Equation (15.2) will not work for a set of points that are scattered. To calculate the slope of the **line of best fit** running through a set of scattered points, a procedure is needed that gives the **average slope**, taking into account the values for all of the points. The equation for calculating the b, the slope of the regression line, is:

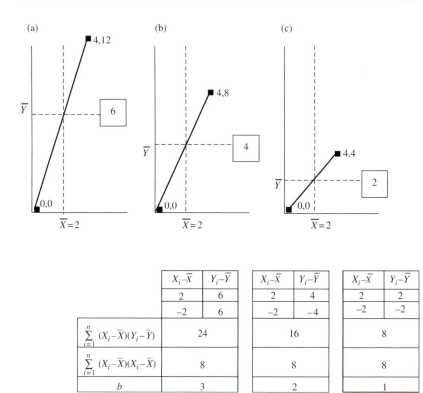

Figure 15.4 Graphs (a), (b), and (c) show three lines of slope 3, 2, and 1 respectively, with two data points on each. The six points have been combined in (d), and the line of best fit through these would be expected to have a slope of 2.0. Use of equation (15.3) gives this appropriate average for b.

$$b = \frac{\displaystyle\sum_{i=1}^{n} (X_i - \bar{X})(Y_i - \bar{Y})}{\displaystyle\sum_{i=1}^{n} (X_i - \bar{X})(X_i - \bar{X})} \tag{15.3}$$

This is an extension of equation (15.2). Instead of calculating the change in X and Y from any two data points, equation (15.3) calculates an average slope using every point in the data set.

First, the means of X and Y are separately calculated. Then, for each data point, the value of X minus its mean is multiplied by the value of Y minus its

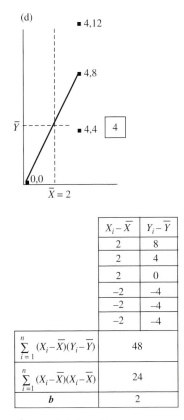

Figure 15.4 (Cont.)

mean and these values summed. This is the numerator of equation (15.3), which is then divided by the sum of each value of X minus its mean and squared.

It is easy to see how equation (15.3) will give an appropriate average value for the slope. The first examples are for points that lie on straight lines.

For a line with a slope of +1, as X increases by one unit from its mean, the value of Y will also increase by one unit from its mean (and *vice versa* if X decreases). The difference between any value of X and its mean will always be the same as the difference between any value of Y and its mean, so the numerator and denominator of equation (15.3) will be the same, thus giving a b value of 1.0 (Figure 15.3(a)).

For a line with a slope of +3, as X increases by one unit from its mean, the value of Y will increase by three units from its mean (and *vice versa* if X decreases). Therefore, the value of the numerator of equation (15.3) will always be three times the size of the denominator, no matter how many points are included, thus giving a b value of 3.0 (Figure 15.3(b)).

For a line with a slope of -1, as X increases by one unit from its mean, the value of Y will decrease by one unit from its mean (and *vice versa* if X decreases). Therefore the numerator of equation (15.3) will give a total that is the same magnitude but the negative of the denominator, thus giving a b value of -1.0 (Figure 15.3(c)).

For a line with a slope of -3, as X increases by one unit from its mean, the value of Y will decrease by three units from its mean (and *vice versa* if X decreases), so the numerator of equation (15.3) will always have a negative sign and be three times the value of the denominator, thus giving a b value of -3.0.

Finally, for a line running parallel to the X axis, every value of $Y_i - \bar{Y}$ will be zero, so the total of the numerator of equation (15.3) will also be zero, thus giving a b value of zero (Figure 15.3(d)).

When the data are scattered, equation (15.3) will also give the **average** change in Y in relation to the increase in X. Figure 15.4 gives an example. First, cases 15.4(a), (b), and (c) show three lines, each of which has been drawn through two data points. These lines have slopes of 3.0, 2.0, and 1.0, respectively, and the calculation of each b value is given in the box under the graph. In Figure 15.4(d) the six data points have been combined. Intuitively, this group of six scattered points should have a slope of 2.0, since this is the average of the slopes of the three lines shown in (a), (b), and (c). Equation (15.3) gives this value.

15.4   Calculation of the intercept with the *Y* axis

The intercept of the regression line with the Y axis when $X = 0$ is easy to calculate, using an extension of the formula for the regression line.

Since:

$$Y = a + bX \qquad\qquad (15.4) \text{ copied from } (15.1)$$

then:

$$\bar{Y} = a + b\bar{X} \qquad\qquad (15.5)$$

which can be rearranged to give the value of a from:

$$a = \bar{Y} - b\bar{X} \qquad\qquad (15.6)$$

and statistical packages will do this as part of a regression analysis.

15.5 Testing the significance of the slope and the intercept of the regression line

Although the equation for a regression line describes the functional relationship between X and Y, it does not show whether the slope of the line and the intercept are significantly different to zero.

For a population, the equation of the line of best fit is:

$$Y = \alpha + \beta X \qquad\qquad (15.7)$$

but, since life scientists usually only have data for a sample, the population statistics α and β are only estimated by the sample statistics a and b. Therefore you need to test the null hypotheses that a and b are from a population where α and β are zero. (Please note that you will find different symbols for the intercept and slope in some texts. Introductory texts generally use a and b (and for a population α and β) for the intercept and slope, but more advanced texts use b_0 and b_1 for these two sample statistics and β_0 and β_1 for the equivalent population statistics. Here I have used the same symbols as most introductory texts for clarity.)

15.5.1 Testing the hypothesis that the slope is significantly different to zero

One method for testing whether the slope of a regression line is significantly different to a slope of zero is very similar to the one factor ANOVA described in Chapter 9. A pictorial explanation is given in Figures 15.5 and 15.6.

Graphs of four regression lines are shown in Figure 15.5, together with a horizontal line showing the average value of Y, which the regression line will always cross. If there is no increase or decrease in the value of Y as X increases, the regression line will have a slope of zero and be indistinguishable from the line showing $\bar{Y}$ (Figure 15.5(a)). Nevertheless, samples taken from a population where β is zero will, by chance, have values of b distributed around zero, often giving regression lines that are slightly tilted upwards or downwards (Figure 15.5 (b) and (c)). Finally, if there is a marked increase or decrease in Y as X increases, the regression line will be strongly tilted (e.g. a negative slope is shown in Figure 15.5(d)).

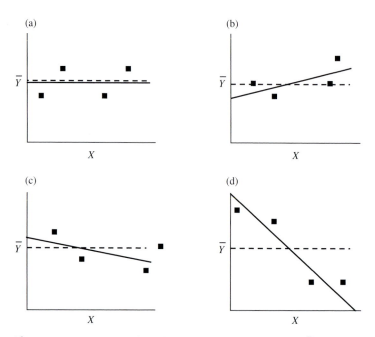

Figure 15.5 A regression line always crosses the line showing $\bar{Y}$. (a) If the slope is exactly zero, the regression line will be indistinguishable from the horizontal line showing $\bar{Y}$. Samples from a population where the slope β is zero will nevertheless be expected to include cases with small (b) positive and (c) negative slopes. (d) If Y increases or decreases markedly as X increases, the regression line will be strongly tilted from the line showing $\bar{Y}$. A negative slope is shown as an example.

The amount by which the regression line is tilted from the horizontal can be detected in the same way a one factor ANOVA detects whether several treatment means are all similar to the grand mean, or whether any are significantly displaced from it.

In Chapter 9 it was described how a one factor ANOVA calculates an F ratio by dividing the mean square for treatment (i.e. treatment + error) by the mean square for error only. If treatment has no effect, the treatment means will be the same or close to the grand mean, so the F ratio will be close to 1.0. The test for whether the slope of a regression line is significantly different to the horizontal line showing $\bar{Y}$ is done in a similar way.

First, the regression line will be tilted from the line showing $\bar{Y}$ because of **the variation explained by the regression equation (regression plus error)**.

Second, each of the points in the scatter plot will be displaced upwards or downwards from the regression line **because of the remaining variation (error only)**.

It is easy to calculate the sums of squares and mean squares for these two separate sources of variation. Figure 15.6 shows scatter plots for two sets of data. The first regression line (15.6(a)) has a large positive slope and the second (15.6(b)) has a slope much closer to zero. The horizontal line on each graph shows $\bar{Y}$.

Here you need to think about the vertical displacement of each point from the line showing $\bar{Y}$. To illustrate this, the point at the top far right of each scatter plot in Figure 15.6 has been identified by a circle instead of a square.

The vertical arrow running up from $\bar{Y}$ to each of the circled points $(Y - \bar{Y})$ indicates the **total variation** or displacement of that point from $\bar{Y}$. This distance can be partitioned into the two sources of variation mentioned above.

The first is the amount of displacement **explained by the regression line (which is affected by both the regression plus error)** and is the distance $(\hat{Y} - \bar{Y})$ shown by the heavy part of the vertical arrow in Figure 15.6.

The second is the distance $(Y - \hat{Y})$ shown by the lighter vertical part of the arrow in Figure 15.6. This is **unexplained variation** or **error** and often called the **residual variation**, since it is the amount of variation remaining between the data points and $\bar{Y}$ that cannot be explained by the regression line.

This gives a way of calculating an F ratio that indicates how much of the variation can be accounted for by the regression.

First, you can calculate the sum of squares for the variation explained by the regression line by squaring the vertical distance between the regression line and $\bar{Y}$ for each point $(\hat{Y} - \bar{Y})$ and adding these together. Dividing this sum of squares by the appropriate number of degrees of freedom will give the mean square due to explained variation (regression plus error).

Second, you can calculate the sum of squares for the unexplained variation by squaring the vertical distance between each point and the regression line $(Y - \hat{Y})$ and adding these together. Dividing this sum of squares by the appropriate number of degrees of freedom will give the mean square due to unexplained variation or 'error'.

At this stage, you have sums of squares and mean squares for two sources of variation that will be very familiar to you from the explanation of one factor ANOVA in Chapter 9:

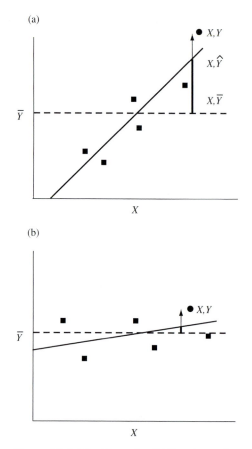

(a)

(b)

Figure 15.6 The diagonal solid line shows the regression through a scatter plot of six points, and the dashed horizontal line shows $\bar{Y}$. The vertical arrow shows the displacement of one point, symbolised by a circle instead of a square, from $\bar{Y}$. The distance between the point and the Y average $(Y - \bar{Y})$ is the total variation, which can be partitioned into variation explained by the regression line and unexplained variation or error. The heavy part of the vertical line $(\hat{Y} - \bar{Y})$ shows the displacement explained by the regression line (regression plus error) and the remainder $(Y - \hat{Y})$ is unexplained variation (error). Note that (a) when the slope is large the explained component is also large, and (b) when the slope is close to zero the explained component is very small.

(a) **The variation explained by the regression line (regression plus error).**

(b) **The unexplained residual variation (error only).**

Therefore, to get an F ratio that shows the proportion of the variation explained by the **regression line compared with the unexplained variation due to error, you divide the mean square for (a) by the mean square for (b).**

$$F_{1,n-2} = \frac{MS \text{ regression}}{MS \text{ residual}} \qquad (15.8)$$

If the regression line has a slope close to zero (Figure 15.5(a)), both the numerator and denominator of equation (15.5) will be similar, so the value of the F statistic will be approximately 1.0. As the slope of the line increases (Figure 15.5(b), (c), and (d)), the numerator of equation (15.5) will become larger, so the value of F will also increase. As F increases, the probability that the data have been taken from a population where the slope of the regression line, β, is zero will decrease and will eventually be less than 0.05. Most statistical packages will calculate the F statistic and give the probability. There is an explanation for the number of degrees of freedom for the F ratio in Box 15.1.

Box 15.1 A note on the number of degrees of freedom in an ANOVA of the slope of the regression line

The example in Section 15.6 includes an ANOVA table with an F statistic and probability for the significance of the slope of the regression line (Table 15.3). Note that the 'regression' mean square, which is equivalent to the 'treatment' mean square in a single factor ANOVA, has only one degree of freedom. This is the case for **any** regression analysis, despite the sample size used for the analysis. In contrast, for a single factor ANOVA the number of degrees of freedom is one less than the number of treatments. This difference needs explaining.

For a single factor ANOVA, all but one of the treatment means are **free to vary**, but the value of the 'final' one is constrained because the grand mean is a set value. Therefore, the number of degrees of freedom for the treatment mean square is always one less than the number of treatments.

In contrast, for any regression line every value of $\hat{Y}$ must (by definition) lie on the line. For a regression line of known slope, once the first value of $\hat{Y}$ has been plotted the remainder are no longer **free to vary** since they must lie on the line, so the regression mean square has only one degree of freedom.

The degrees of freedom for error in a single factor ANOVA are the sum of one less than the number within each of the treatments. Since a degree of freedom is lost for every treatment, if there are a total of n replicates (the sum of the replicates in all treatments) and k treatments, the error degrees of freedom are $n - k$. In contrast, the degrees of freedom for the residual (error) variation in a regression analysis are always $n - 2$. This is because a regression line, which only ever has one degree of freedom, is always only equivalent to an experiment with two treatments.

15.5.2 Testing whether the intercept of the regression line is significantly different to zero

The value for the intercept a calculated from a sample is only an estimate of the population statistic α. Consequently, a positive or negative value of a might be obtained in a sample from a population where α is zero. The standard deviation of the points scattered around the regression line can be used to calculate the 95% confidence interval for a, and a single sample t test can be used to compare the value of a to zero or any other expected value. Once again, most statistical packages include a test of whether a differs significantly from zero.

15.5.3 The coefficient of determination r^2

The coefficient of determination, symbolised by r^2, is a statistic that shows the **proportion of the total variation of the values of Y from the average $\bar{Y}$ that is explained by the regression line**. It is the regression sum of squares divided by the total sum of squares:

$$r^2 = \frac{\text{Sum of squares explained by the regression ((a) above)}}{\text{Total sum of squares ((a) + (b) above)}} \quad (15.9)$$

which will only ever be a number from zero to 1.0. If the points all lie along the regression line and it has a slope that is different to zero, the unexplained

Table 15.1. Data for the age of a person and the number of mites found on 50 of their eyelashes

Age (years)	Number of mites
3	5
6	13
9	16
12	14
15	18
18	23
21	20
24	32
27	29
30	28

component (quantity (b)) will be zero and r^2 will be 1. If the explained sum of squares is small in relation to the unexplained, r^2 will be a small number.

15.6 An example – mites that live in your hair follicles

The follicle mite *Demodex folliculorum* is less than a millimetre long and lives in the hair follicles of humans, including those of the eyelashes. A fascinating account of the ecology of these mites, including illustrations, can be found in Andrews (1976), who notes that most adult humans have *D. folliculorum* living in the hair follicles of the 'chin, the nose, or the forehead and scalp'. These mites are acquired after birth and prefer follicles where a relatively large amount of sebum (the waxy material produced by the sebaceous gland within the follicle) is produced. A biomedical scientist hypothesised that the number of mites would be determined by a person's age. To test this they obtained ten volunteers, plucked 25 eyelashes at random from each eye and counted the number of mites. These bivariate data for age in years and the number of mites are in Table 15.1.

From a regression analysis of these data a statistical package would give values for the equation for the regression line, plus a test of the hypotheses that the intercept, a, and slope, b, are from a population where α and β are zero.

Table 15.2. An example of the table of results from a regression analysis. The value of the intercept a (5.733) is given in the first row, labelled '(Constant)' under the heading 'Value'. The slope b (0.853) is given in the second row (labelled as the independent variable 'Age') under the heading 'Value'. The final two columns give the results of t tests comparing a and b to zero. These show the intercept, a, is significantly different to zero ($P = 0.035$) and the slope b is also significantly different to zero ($P = 0.001$)

Model	Value	Std error	t	Significance
Constant	5.733	2.265	2.531	0.035
Age	0.853	0.122	7.006	0.001

Table 15.3. An example of the results of an analysis of the slope of a regression. The significant F ratio shows the slope is significantly different to zero

	Sum of squares	df	Mean square	F	Significance
Regression	539.6481	1	539.648	49.086	0.000
Residual	87.952	8	10.994		
Total	627.600	9			

The output would be similar in format to Table 15.2.

From the results in Table 15.2 the equation for the regression line is mites $= 5.773 + 0.853 \times$ age. The slope is significantly different to zero (in this case it is positive) and the intercept is also significantly different to zero. You could use the regression equation to predict the number of mites on a person of any age between 3 and 30.

Most statistical packages will give an ANOVA of the slope. For the data in Table 15.1 there is a significant relationship between mite numbers and age (Table 15.3).

Finally, the value of r^2 is also given. Sometimes there are two values: r^2, which is the statistic for the sample, and a value called 'Adjusted r^2', which is an estimate for the population from which the sample has been taken. The r^2 value is usually the one reported in the results of the regression. For the example above you would get the following values:

$$r = 0.927, \quad r^2 = 0.860, \quad \text{adjusted } r^2 = 0.842$$

This shows that 86% of the variation in mite numbers with age can be predicted by the regression line.

15.7 Predicting a value of *Y* from a value of *X*

Since the regression line has the average slope through a set of scattered points, the predicted value of *Y* is only the **average** expected for a given value of *X*. If the r^2 value is 1.0, the value of *Y* will be predicted without error, since all the data points will lie on the regression line. Usually, however, the points will be scattered around the line. More advanced texts (e.g. Sokal and Rohlf (1995), Zar (1999)) describe how you can calculate the 95% confidence interval for a value of *Y* and thus predict its likely range.

15.8 Predicting a value of *X* from a value of *Y*

Often you might want to estimate a value of the independent variable *X* from the dependent variable *Y*. Here is an example.

The concentration of sugar in fruit can only be directly measured by damaging the fruit, which makes it unsuitable for sale. Sugar content varies among fruit from the same plant and from the same farm, and fruit relatively high in sugar usually taste sweeter and can often be sold for a higher price. Therefore it would be advantageous to identify fruit with the highest sugar concentration without damaging them before sale. It has been shown that the amount of infra red light reflected from the surface of certain fruit, such as melons and tomatoes, is significantly dependent on the sugar concentration. Therefore, if sugar concentration could be predicted from the amount of infra red light reflected from the fruit, it would provide a way of estimating sugar concentration without damage.

In this case it is **not** appropriate to designate sugar concentration as the dependent variable and calculate a regression equation, because it clearly does not depend on the amount of infra red light reflected from the fruit, so one of the assumptions of regression would be violated.

Predicting *X* from *Y* can be done by rearranging the regression equation for any point from:

$$Y_i = a + bX_i \qquad\qquad (15.10)$$

to:

$$X_i = \frac{Y_i - a}{b} \qquad\qquad (15.11)$$

but here too the 95% confidence interval around the estimated value of X must also be calculated, because the measurement of Y is likely to include some error. Methods for doing this are given in more advanced texts (e.g. Sokal and Rohlf, 1995).

15.9 The danger of extrapolating beyond the range of data available

Although regression analysis draws a line of best fit through a set of data, it is dangerous to make predictions beyond the measured range of X. Figure 15.7 illustrates that a predicted regression line may not be a correct estimation of the value of Y outside this range.

15.10 Assumptions of linear regression analysis

The procedure for linear regression analysis described in this chapter is often described as a Model I regression, and makes several assumptions.

First, the values of Y are assumed to be from a population of values normally distributed about the regression line. If this does not apply, a regression analysis should not be used. More advanced texts discuss methods for testing this assumption.

Second, it is assumed the independent variable X is measured without error. In practice, it is often difficult to ensure this and many texts note that X should be measured with little error. For example, levels of an independent variable determined by the experimenter, such as several different temperature treatments, are usually measured with very little error indeed. In contrast, a variable such as the wet weight of a frog is likely to be measured with a great deal of error. When the dependent variable is subject to error, a different analysis called Model II regression is appropriate. Again, this is described in more advanced texts.

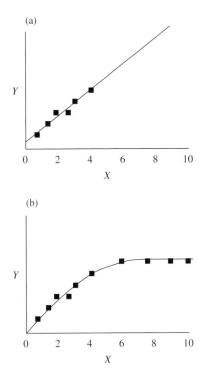

Figure 15.7 It is risky to use a regression line to extrapolate values of Y beyond the measured range of X. The regression line (a) based on the data for values of X ranging from 1 to 5 does not necessarily give an accurate prediction (b) of the values of Y beyond that range.

Third, it is assumed that the dependent variable is determined by the independent variable. This was discussed in Section 14.2.

Fourth, the relationship between X and Y is assumed to be linear and it is important to be confident of this before carrying out the analysis. A scatter plot of the data should be drawn to look for any obvious departures from linearity. In some cases it may be possible to transform the Y variable (see Chapter 12) to give a linear relationship and proceed with a regression analysis on the transformed data.

Finally, the variance of the Y values is also assumed to be the same, whatever the value of X. Tests for heteroscedasticity in regression are described in more advanced texts, but again a scatter plot may reveal if the variance of the points around the regression line is similar across the range of X. If not, transformation of the Y variable may remedy this problem.

15.11   Further topics in regression

This chapter is an introduction to linear regression analysis. More advanced analyses include procedures for comparing the slopes and intercepts of two or more regression lines. Non-linear regression models can be fitted to data where the relationship between X and Y is exponential, logarithmic, or even more complex. Multiple linear regression is used to separate the effects of several independent variables upon a dependent variable. These topics are beyond the scope of this book but the understanding of simple linear regression developed here will make them easier to understand if you need to use them.

16 | Non-parametric statistics

16.1   Introduction

Parametric tests are designed for analysing data from a known distribution, and the majority assume a normally distributed population. Although parametric tests are quite robust to departures from normality, and major ones can often be reduced by transformation, there are some cases where the population is so grossly non-normal that parametric testing is unwise. In these cases a powerful analysis can often still be done by using a **non-parametric** test.

Non-parametric tests are not just alternatives to the parametric procedures for analysing ratio, interval, and ordinal data described in Chapters 7 to 15. Often life scientists obtain data that have been measured on a nominal scale. For example, Table 3.3 gave the numbers of basal cell carcinomas detected and removed from different areas of the human body. This is a sample containing frequencies in several discrete and mutually exclusive categories and there are non-parametric tests for analysing these types of data (Chapter 17).

16.2   The danger of assuming normality when a population is grossly non-normal

Most parametric tests have been specifically designed for analysing data from populations having bell-shaped distributions with 66.27% of values occurring within $\mu \pm 1$ standard deviation and 95% within $\mu \pm 1.96$ standard deviations (Chapter 6). This distribution is used to determine the range within which 95% of the values of the sample mean, $\bar{X}$, will occur when samples of a particular size are taken from a population. If $\bar{X}$ occurs outside the range of $\mu \pm 1.96$, the probability the sample has come from

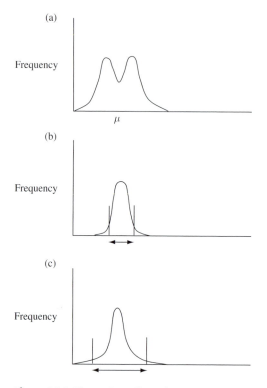

Figure 16.1 Illustration of how the range in which the means of samples from a grossly non-normal population does not correspond to the expected range, assuming the population is normally distributed. (a) Distribution of a bimodal population, (b) Actual shape of the distribution of means of sample size $n = 30$ from the population shown in (a). (c) Shape of the distribution of means calculated from the standard error when $n = 30$, assuming the population is normally distributed. Horizontal arrows show the range within which 95% of means would be expected to occur. Note that the expected range in (c) is much wider than the true range in (b).

that population is less than 5%. If the population is not normally distributed, the range occupied by 95% of the values of the mean may be either wider or narrower than assumed, in which case judgements about statistical significance made on the basis of the normal distribution will be misleading.

An example is shown in Figure 16.1 . The population is bimodal and the range within which 95% of the values of the means of samples of size $n = 30$ from this population actually occur is narrower than the range predicted if the population is assumed to be normally distributed.

16.3   The value of making a preliminary inspection of the data

It has already been emphasised that parametric tests for comparing means can often be applied to data from populations that are not normally distributed, because the distribution of the means of samples from most populations will usually be relatively normal (Chapter 6). Once again, however, the example in Section 16.2 emphasises the value of graphing the data to inspect it for normality and homoscedasticity before attempting a statistical analysis.

The next two chapters describe tests for analysing nominal scale data, followed by some non-parametric alternatives to the parametric tests for independent and related samples described in Chapters 7–11, as well as a non-parametric test for correlation.

17 | Non-parametric tests for nominal scale data

17.1　Introduction

Life scientists often collect samples in which the experimental units can be assigned to two or more discrete and mutually exclusive categories. For example, a sample of 20 humans can be partitioned into the two mutually exclusive categories of 'right-handed' or 'left-handed' (since even people who claim to be ambidextrous still perform a greater proportion of actions with one hand and can be classified as having a dominant right or left hand). These two categories are discrete because there is no intermediate state and mutually exclusive because a person cannot be assigned to both. They also make up the entire set of possible outcomes within the sample and therefore are contingent upon each other, since for a fixed sample size a decrease in the number in one category must be accompanied by an increase in the number in the other and vice versa.

These are nominal scale data (Chapter 3). The questions researchers ask about these data are the sort asked about any sample(s) from a population.

First, you may want to know the probability a sample has been taken from a population having a known or expected proportion within each category. For example, the proportion of left-handed people in the world is close to 0.1 (10%), which can be considered the proportion in the population, since it is from a sample of several million people. A biomedical scientist, who knew that the proportion of left- and right-handed people showed some variation among occupations, sampled 20 statisticians and found that four were left-handed and 16 right-handed. The question is whether the proportions in the sample were significantly different from the expected proportions of 0.1 and 0.9 respectively. The difference between the population and the sample might be solely due to chance, or also reflect career choice.

Second, you may want to know the probability that two or more samples have come from the same population. For example, a geneticist noticed that the children of male deep-sea divers seemed to be predominantly female. Consequently they sampled 100 male divers and 100 male deckhands within a similar age range and who worked on the same dive boats. For each individual they recorded the gender of their first-born child. The offspring of the divers were 67 females and 33 males, while the offspring of the deckhands were 53 females and 47 males. Here too, the difference between the two samples might be due to chance, or also occupation.

For both of these examples a method is needed that gives the probability of obtaining the observed outcome under the null hypothesis. This chapter describes some tests for analysing samples of categorical data.

17.2   Comparing observed and expected frequencies – the chi-square test for goodness of fit

The chi-square test for goodness of fit compares the observed frequencies in a sample with those expected in a population, and the following example may be familiar to you from an introductory biology course. The genes that control pelt colour in guinea pigs are described as 'dominant' and 'recessive', with the gene for a lack of pigment being recessive to the gene for brown pelt. This is because the dominant gene codes for a protein that makes brown pigment, while the recessive gene does not code for any pigment. Therefore, an individual with two copies of the recessive gene will be albino, but heterozygotes with one copy, and homozygotes with two copies, of the brown gene will be brown. Consequently, you would expect the proportions of three brown to one albino among the offspring from a cross between two heterozygotes. To test this, a geneticist crossed several guinea pigs heterozygous for pelt colour and obtained 100 offspring altogether. Under the null hypothesis the expected numbers in the sample were 75 brown and 25 albino, but the sample actually contained 86 brown and 14 albino offspring. This difference from the expected frequencies in the sample might be due to chance, or because the null hypothesis is incorrect. The chi-square test calculates the probability that a sample has come from a population with the expected proportions in each category.

Table 17.1. A worked example comparing the observed frequencies in a sample to those expected from the proportions in the population. The observed frequencies in a sample of 20 are 4:16 and the expected frequencies are 2:18

Handed	Left	Right
Observed	4	16
Expected	2	18
Obs – Exp	2	−2
$(\text{Obs} - \text{Exp})^2$	4	4
$\dfrac{(\text{Obs} - \text{Exp})^2}{\text{Exp}}$	2	0.22

$$\chi^2 = \sum_{i=1}^{n} \frac{(o_i - e_i)^2}{e_i} = 2.22$$

The chi-square statistic is the sum of each of the observed frequencies, minus its expected frequency, squared, and then divided by the expected frequency:

$$\chi^2 = \sum_{i=1}^{n} \frac{(o_i - e_i)^2}{e_i} \tag{17.1}$$

This is sometimes written as:

$$\chi^2 = \sum_{i=1}^{n} \frac{\left(f_i - \widehat{f_i}\right)^2}{\widehat{f_i}} \tag{17.2}$$

where f_i is the observed frequency and $\widehat{f_i}$ is the expected frequency.

It does not matter whether the difference between the observed and expected frequencies is positive or negative, because the square of any difference will be positive.

If there is perfect agreement between every observed and expected frequency, the value of chi-square will be zero. Nevertheless, even if the null hypothesis applies, samples are unlikely to always contain the exact proportions present in the population. By chance, small departures are likely and larger departures will also occur, all of which will generate positive values of chi-square. The most extreme 5% of departures from the expected ratio are considered statistically significant and will exceed a critical value of chi-square.

Table 17.1 gives a worked example for the sample of left- and right-handed statisticians mentioned above.

The value of chi-square in Table 17.1 has one degree of freedom because the sample size is fixed, so as soon as the frequency of one of the two categories is set the other is no longer free to vary. The 5% critical value of chi-square with one degree of freedom is 3.84, so the proportions of left- and right-handed people in the sample are not significantly different to the expected proportions of 0.1 to 0.9. The chi-square test for goodness of fit can be extended to any number of categories and the degrees of freedom will be $k - 1$ (where k is the number of categories). Statistical packages will calculate the value of chi-square and its probability.

17.2.1 Small sample sizes

When expected frequencies are small, the calculated chi-square statistic is inaccurate and tends to be too large, therefore indicating a lower than appropriate probability, which increases the risk of Type 1 error. It used to be recommended that no expected frequency in a goodness of fit test should be less than five, but this has been relaxed somewhat in the light of more recent research, and it is now recommended that no more than 20% of expected frequencies should be less than five.

An entirely different method, which is not subject to bias when the sample size is small, can be used to analyse these data. It is an example of a group of procedures called **randomisation tests** that will be discussed further in Chapter 18. Instead of calculating a statistic that is used to estimate the probability of an outcome, a randomisation test uses a computer program **to simulate the repeated random sampling of an hypothetical population containing the expected proportions in each category**. These samples will often contain the same proportions as the population, but departures will occur by chance. The simulated sampling is **iterated,** meaning it is repeated, several thousand times and the resultant distribution of the statistic used to identify the most extreme 5% of departures from the expected proportions. Finally, the actual proportions in the real sample are compared with this distribution. If the sample statistic falls within the region where the most extreme 5% of departures from the expected occur, the sample is considered significantly different to the population.

Repeated random sampling of an hypothetical population is an example of a more general procedure called the **Monte Carlo method** that uses the properties of the sample, or the expected properties of a population, and

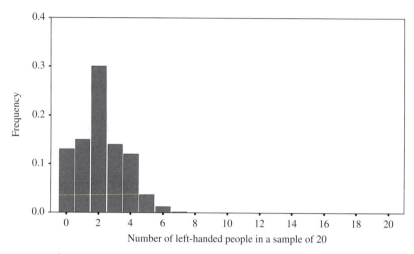

Figure 17.1 An example of the distribution of outcomes from a Monte Carlo simulation, where 10 000 samples of size 20 are taken at random from a population containing 0.1 left-handed and 0.9 right-handed people. Note that the probability of obtaining four or more left-handed people in a sample of 20 is greater than 0.05.

takes a large number of simulated random samples to create a distribution that would apply under the null hypothesis.

For the data in Table 17.1, where the sample size was 20 and the expected proportions were 0.1 left-handers to 0.9 right-handers, a randomisation test works by taking several thousand random samples, each of size 20, from an hypothetical population containing these proportions. This will generate a distribution of outcomes similar to the one shown in Figure 17.1, which is for 10 000 samples. If the procedure is repeated another 10 000 times, the outcome is unlikely to be exactly the same, but nevertheless will be very similar to Figure 17.1, because so many samples have been taken. It is clear from Figure 17.1 that the likelihood of a sample containing four or more people who are left-handed is greater than 0.05.

17.3   Comparing proportions among two or more independent samples

Life scientists often want to compare the proportions in categories among two or more samples to test the null hypothesis that the samples have come from the same population. Unlike the previous example, there are no

Table 17.2. Data for samples of 20 cane toads taken at each of three locations in Queensland, Australia and dissected to see if they were infected with, or free from, intestinal parasites

	Rockhampton	Bowen	Mackay
Infected	12	7	14
Uninfected	8	13	6

expected proportions – instead these tests examine whether the proportions in each category are heterogeneous among samples.

17.3.1 The chi-square test for heterogeneity

Here is an example for three samples, each containing two mutually exclusive categories. The cane toad, *Bufo marinus*, was deliberately introduced to Australia in an attempt to control insect pests of sugar cane, and has since become extremely abundant in northern Queensland. Unfortunately the cane toad is now a pest because it preys on a wide variety of small native species and can poison animals that attack it. The population density of cane toads appears to have peaked and subsequently decreased in some areas of Queensland, so conservation biologists are sampling these in an attempt to find out if the toads are being affected by parasites or pathogens that might be useful as biological control agents. A researcher decided to test the hypothesis that the proportion of cane toads with intestinal parasites was the same in three different areas of Queensland, so they sampled 20 from each area, dissected them, and categorised them as being infected or free from intestinal parasites. The researcher did not have a preconceived hypothesis about the expected proportions of infected and uninfected toads – they simply wanted to compare the three samples. The data are shown in Table 17.2. This format is often called a **contingency table**.

These data are used to calculate an **expected frequency** for each of the six cells. This is done by first calculating the row and column totals (Table 17.3(a)) often called the **marginal totals**. The proportions of infected and uninfected toads in the marginal totals shown in the right-hand column of Table 17.3 are the overall proportions within the sample. Therefore, under the null hypothesis of no difference in the proportions

Table 17.3. (a) The marginal totals for the data in Table 17.2. To obtain the expected frequency for any cell, its row and column total are multiplied together and divided by the grand total. (b) Note that the expected frequencies at each location (11:9) are the same and also correspond to the proportions of the marginal totals (33:27)

	Rockhampton	Bowen	Mackay	Row totals
(a) Observed frequencies and marginal totals				
Infected	12	7	14	33
Uninfected	8	13	6	27
Column totals	20	20	20	Grand total = 60
(b) Expected frequencies calculated from the marginal totals				
Infected	11	11	11	33
Uninfected	9	9	9	27
Column totals	20	20	20	Grand total = 60

among locations, each will have the same proportion of infected toads. To obtain the expected frequency for any cell under the null hypothesis, the column total and the row total corresponding to that cell are multiplied together and divided by the grand total. For example, in Table 17.3(b) the expected frequency of infected toads in a sample of 20 from Rockhampton is $(20 \times 33) \div 60 = 11$ and the expected frequency of uninfected toads from Mackay is $(20 \times 27) \div 60 = 9$.

After the expected frequencies have been calculated for all cells, equation (17.1) is used to calculate the chi-square statistic. The number of degrees of freedom for this analysis is one less than the number of columns, multiplied by one less than the number of rows, since all but one of the values within each column and each row are free to vary, but the final one is not because of the fixed marginal total. Here, therefore, the number of degrees of freedom is $2 \times 1 = 2$. The smallest contingency table possible has two rows and two columns (this is called a 2×2 table), which will give a chi-square statistic with only one degree of freedom.

17.3.2 The G test or log-likelihood ratio

The **G test** or **log-likelihood ratio** is another way of estimating the chi-square statistic. The formula for the G statistic is:

$$G = 2 \sum_{i=1}^{n} f_i \ln \left(\frac{f_i}{\hat{f}_i} \right)$$ (17.3)

This means, 'The G statistic is twice the sum of the frequency of each cell multiplied by the natural logarithm of each observed frequency divided by the expected frequency.' This formula will give a statistic of zero when each expected frequency is equal to its observed frequency, but any discrepancy will give a positive value of G. Some statisticians recommend the G test and others recommend the chi-square test. There is a summary of tests recommended for categorical data near the end of this chapter.

17.3.3 Randomisation tests for contingency tables

A randomisation test procedure similar to the one discussed in Section 17.2.1 for goodness of fit tests can be used for any contingency table. First, the marginal totals of the table are calculated and give the expected proportions when there is no difference among samples. Then the Monte Carlo method is used to repeatedly 'sample' an hypothetical population containing these proportions with the constraint that both the column and row totals are fixed. Randomisation tests are available in some statistical packages.

17.4   Bias when there is one degree of freedom

When there is only one degree of freedom and the total sample size is less than 200, the calculated value of chi-square has been shown to be inaccurate because it is too large. Consequently it gives a probability that is smaller than appropriate, thus increasing the risk of Type 1 error. This bias increases as sample size decreases, so the following formula, called **Yates' correction** or **the continuity correction**, was designed to improve the accuracy of the chi-square statistic for small samples with one degree of freedom.

Yates' correction removes 0.5 from the **absolute** difference between each observed and expected frequency. (The absolute difference is used because it converts all differences to positive numbers, which will be reduced by subtracting 0.5. Otherwise, any negative values of $o_i - e_i$ would have to be increased by 0.5 to make their absolute size and the square of that smaller.) The absolute value is the positive of any number and is indicated by enclosing the number or its symbol by two vertical bars (e.g. $|-6| = 6$). The subscript 'adj' after the value of chi-square means it has been adjusted by Yates' correction.

$$\chi^2_{adj} = \sum_{i=1}^{n} \frac{(|o_i - e_i| - 0.5)^2}{e_i} \tag{17.4}$$

From equation (17.4) it is clear that the compensatory effect of Yates' correction will become less and less as sample size increases. Some authors (e.g. Zar, 1999) recommend that Yates' correction is applied to all chi-square tests having only one degree of freedom, but others suggest it is unnecessary for large samples and recommend the use of the Fisher Exact Test (see Section 17.4.1 below) for smaller ones.

17.4.1 The Fisher Exact Test for 2×2 tables

The Fisher Exact Test accurately calculates the probability that two samples, each containing two categories, are from the same population. **This test is not subject to bias** and is recommended when sample sizes are small or more than 20% of expected frequencies are less than five, but it can be used for any 2×2 contingency table.

The Fisher Exact Test is unusual in that it does not calculate a statistic that is used to estimate the probability of a departure from the null hypothesis. Instead, the probability is calculated directly.

The easiest way to explain the Fisher Exact Test is with an example. Table 17.4 gives data for the presence or absence of a lizard called the banded gecko on ten western Pacific islands. An examination of museum specimens showed that this lizard was present on most islands in the western Pacific in the mid-nineteenth century, but since then the vegetation of many has been cleared for agriculture. A conservation biologist, who was interested in whether vegetation clearing had any effect on the presence of the banded gecko, sampled five islands that had been cleared and five that had not. The results for the presence or lack of detection of the banded gecko are in Table 17.4. These frequencies are too small for accurate analysis using a chi-square test.

If there were no effect of clearing you would expect, under the null hypothesis, that the proportions of islands with geckos in each sample (cleared and uncleared) would be the same as the marginal totals

Table 17.4. Data for the presence of the banded gecko on a sample of ten islands in the western Pacific. The sample deliberately included five islands that had been cleared for agriculture and five that had not. The marginal totals show that four islands have geckos present and six do not

	Island cleared for agriculture	Island not cleared	
Banded gecko present	0	4	4
Banded gecko not found	5	1	6
	5	5	10

Table 17.5. Under the null hypothesis that there is no effect of clearing on the banded gecko, the expected proportions of islands with and without geckos in each sample (2:3 and 2:3) will correspond to the marginal totals for the two rows (4:6). The proportions of islands cleared and uncleared (2:2) and (3:3) will also correspond to the marginal totals for the two columns (5:5)

	Island cleared for agriculture	Island not cleared	
Banded gecko present	2	2	4
Banded gecko not found	3	3	6
	5	5	10

(Table 17.5), with any departures being due to chance. The Fisher Exact Test uses the following procedure to calculate the probability of an outcome equal to or more extreme than the one observed, which can be used to decide whether it is statistically significant.

First, the four marginal totals are calculated, as shown in Table 17.5.

Second, all of the possible ways in which the data can be arranged within the four cells of the 2 × 2 table are listed, subject to the constraint that the marginal totals must remain unchanged. This is **the total set of possible outcomes for the sample**. For these marginal totals, the most likely outcome under the null hypothesis of no difference between the samples is shown in Table 17.5 and identified as (c) in Table 17.6.

For a sample of ten islands, five of which must be cleared and five of which must not, together with the constraint that six islands must have geckos

Table 17.6. The total set of possible outcomes for the number of islands with and without banded geckos, subject to the constraint that there are five islands in each of the two groups and four islands have banded geckos present while six do not. The most likely outcome, where the proportions are the same in both types of islands, is shown in the central box (c). The actual outcome is case (e)

	Cleared	Not cleared	Cleared	Not cleared	Cleared	Not cleared	Cleared	Not cleared	Cleared	Not cleared
Gecko present	4	0	3	1	2	2	1	3	0	4
Gecko absent	1	5	2	4	3	3	4	2	5	1
	(a)		(b)		(c) Expected under the null hypothesis		(d)		(e) Observed outcome	

present and four must not, there are five possible outcomes (Table 17.6). To obtain these you start with the outcome expected under the null hypothesis (c), choose one of the four cells (it does not matter which), and add one to that cell. Next, adjust the values in the other three cells so the marginal totals do not change. Continue with this procedure until the number within the cell you have chosen cannot be increased any further without affecting the marginal totals. Then go back to the expected outcome and repeat the procedure by subtracting one from the same cell until the number in it cannot decrease any further without affecting the marginal totals (Table 17.6).

Third, the actual outcome is identified within the total set of possible outcomes. For this example, it is case (e) in Table 17.6. The probability of this outcome, together with any more extreme departures in the same direction from the one expected under the null hypothesis (here there are none more extreme than (e)) can be calculated from the probability of getting this particular arrangement within the four cells by sampling a set of ten islands, four of which contain geckos and six of which do not, with five out of ten cleared. This is similar to the example used to introduce hypothesis testing in Chapter 5, where you had to imagine a sample of beads drawn from a sack. Here, however, a very small group is sampled without replacement, so the initial probability of selecting an island with geckos present is 4/10, but, if one is drawn, the probability of next drawing an island with geckos is now 3/9 (and 6/9 without). I deliberately have not given this calculation because it is long and tedious, and most statistical packages do it as part of the Fisher Exact Test.

The calculation gives the exact probability of getting the observed outcome or a more extreme departure in the same direction from that expected under the null hypothesis. This is a one-tailed probability, since the outcomes in the opposite direction (e.g. on the left of (c) in Table 17.6) have been ignored. For a two-tailed hypothesis you need to double the probability. Once the probability is less than 0.05, the outcome is considered statistically significant.

17.5   Three-dimensional contingency tables

The contingency tables described in this chapter are two dimensional, but three-dimensional tables can also be analysed. For example, if you had two or more samples within which two categorical variables have been measured on each individual (e.g. a person's sex and whether they are left or right-handed), these would give a contingency table consisting of a three-dimensional block of cells with one column and two rows. Three-dimensional chi-square analyses are described in more advanced texts.

17.6   Inappropriate use of tests for goodness of fit and heterogeneity

Tests for goodness of fit and contingency tables assume that the data are mutually exclusive and contingent upon one another. It is also assumed that the categories are the entire set possible within each sample. Occasionally, however, these tests are misused. The most common misuse occurs when samples are incorrectly considered as categories, as shown in the following example.

Marine ecologists often use small traps baited with dead or damaged fish or crustaceans to sample benthic scavengers, such as whelks. A researcher was interested in comparing the numbers of the scavenging whelk *Nassarius subtidalis* in traps baited with four different baits (crab, oyster, fish, and prawn), so they placed one trap containing each bait, plus an empty trap as a control, on the seabed in an area where *N. subtidalis* was common. The traps were left for six hours, retrieved, and the number of *N. subtidalis* inside them counted (Table 17.7).

Fifty whelks were trapped. The data were analysed using a chi-square test for goodness of fit, with the null hypothesis that equal numbers of whelks (in this case 10, since 50 were caught in total and there were five traps) would be expected in each trap.

Unfortunately these data are not suitable for a goodness of fit test, because the five treatments are neither mutually exclusive nor contingent categories within a sample. This is clear if you consider that a whelk that did not enter a particular trap would not **have** to enter another. The numbers in each trap are actually single samples from each treatment.

In contrast, if the whelks caught within each trap were subdivided into the mutually exclusive categories of male and female, it would be appropriate to use a test for heterogeneity to test the (very different) hypothesis that the sex ratio does not vary among treatments, because the two sexes are mutually exclusive and contingent categories within each treatment (Table 17.8). To avoid the pitfall of confusing categories and samples, you need to ask yourself, 'Do I have data for categories that are mutually exclusive and contingent within each sample, or are my "categories" really separate independent samples?'

Table 17.7. Data for the number of *N. subtidalis* found in five traps, four of which contained different baits and one left empty as a control, after six hours. The numbers in each trap are not mutually exclusive or contingent upon the numbers within any other, so the data are unsuitable for analysis by a goodness of fit test

	Crab	Oyster	Fish	Prawn	Control
Number of *N. subtidalis* present	14	1	16	17	2

Table 17.8. Data for the number of *N. subtidalis* found in five traps after six hours. The numbers of male and female whelks in each trap are mutually exclusive and contingent categories, so these data are suitable for a contingency table analysis comparing the proportions of each sex among bait types

	Crab	Oyster	Fish	Prawn	Control
Male	6	1	7	7	0
Female	8	0	9	10	2

17.7   Recommended tests for categorical data

Several tests have been developed for data that are frequencies in mutually exclusive and contingent categories. The following are broad recommendations.

When comparing the frequencies in two or more categories within a single sample to their expected proportions, chi-square can be used where no more than 20% of expected frequencies are less than five. A randomisation test can be used for any sized sample.

For 2 × 2 contingency tables the Fisher Exact Test will give an unbiased probability and is available in most statistical packages.

For contingency tables with more than two rows and columns, the chi-square or *G* test can be used if no more than 20% of expected frequencies are less than five. A randomisation test will give an unbiased probability for any sized sample.

17.8   Comparing proportions among two or more related samples of nominal scale data

If you have measured the same variable more than once on each experimental unit, the samples are not independent and need to be analysed using a test for related samples. Table 17.9 gives an example of two **related** samples of nominal scale data from a laboratory experiment where 12 individually numbered banded geckos were placed in an arena with a background tiled as an alternating 'checkerboard' pattern of large black and white squares. One hour later the background type (black or white) occupied by each lizard was recorded. Next, the silhouette of a predatory bird known to eat banded geckos was displayed above the arena and the background occupied by each lizard recorded a second time. The null hypothesis was that geckos would show no change in the background occupied before and after the sight of the predator, while the alternate hypothesis was that they would change to either a darker or lighter background. It is not appropriate to analyse these data with a test that compares two independent samples.

The **McNemar test for the significance of changes** compares two related samples of nominal scale data in two categories. The data in Table 17.9 are

Table 17.9. The background occupied by 12 banded geckos before and after being exposed to the silhouette of a predatory bird. B = black background, W = white background. These two samples are not independent since they contain the same 12 lizards

Gecko number	Before	After
1	B	B
2	B	B
3	W	B
4	B	B
5	W	B
6	W	W
7	B	B
8	W	B
9	B	B
10	W	B
11	W	B
12	W	B

Table 17.10. The numbers of banded geckos on black and white backgrounds before and after exposure to the silhouette of a predatory bird. Two cells show the individuals whose background preference changed and these are (b) from black to white and (c) from white to black

	After	
Before	Black	White
Black	(a) 5	(b) 0
White	(c) 6	(d) 1

summarised in a 2×2 table giving the number of individuals in all four possible combinations of categories and samples. These are (a) black before and after, (b) black before and white after, (c) white before and black after, and (d) white before and white after (Table 17.10).

The null hypothesis predicts that there will be no difference in the proportions of lizards on each background between the two samples, while the alternate predicts there will be a difference. Therefore, under the null hypothesis, the set of lizards that **did** change backgrounds (combinations (b) and (c)) would be expected to include equal numbers that changed from black to white and from white to black, so you would expect cells (b) and (c) of Table 17.10 to contain equal frequencies. If, however, the background preference differed before and after exposure to the silhouette, the frequencies in these two cells would be expected to be unequal.

In this example six lizards changed backgrounds, so three would be expected to change from black to white and vice versa. The McNemar test ignores categories (a) and (d) where no change has occurred and compares the observed and expected frequencies in cells (b) and (c) using a goodness of fit test (e.g. the chi-square, exact, or randomisation tests for two mutually exclusive categories discussed earlier in this chapter, or the exact probability calculated from the binomial distribution discussed in Chapter 5). If there is a statistically significant difference between the numbers in each of these two categories, it indicates a change between the two samples.

For three or more related samples of nominal scale data in two categories, the **Cochran Q test** is an extension of the McNemar test. These tests are also included in most statistical packages.

18 | Non-parametric tests for ratio, interval, or ordinal scale data

18.1   Introduction

This chapter describes some non-parametric tests for ratio, interval, or ordinal scale data. Non-parametric tests do not use the predictable distribution of sample means, which is the basis of most parametric tests, to infer whether samples are from the same population. Consequently non-parametric tests are generally not as powerful as their parametric equivalents, but, if the data are **grossly** non-normal and cannot be satisfactorily improved by transformation, it is necessary to use a non-parametric test.

Non-parametric tests are often called 'distribution free tests' but most nevertheless assume that the samples being analysed are from populations with the same distribution. **Therefore, most non-parametric tests should not be used where there are gross differences in distribution (including the variance) among samples.** The general rule that the ratio of the largest to smallest sample variance should not exceed 4:1 discussed in Chapter 12 also applies to non-parametric tests.

Many non-parametric tests for ratio, interval, or ordinal data calculate a statistic from a comparison of two or more samples and work in the following way.

First, the raw data are converted to **ranks**. For example, the lowest value is assigned the rank of '1', the next highest '2' etc. This transforms the data to an ordinal scale (see Chapter 3) with the ranks indicating only their relative order. Under the null hypothesis that the samples are from the same population you would expect a similar range of ranks within each, with differences among samples only occurring by chance.

Second, a statistic that reflects any differences in the ranks among samples is calculated and its value compared with the expected distribution of this statistic when samples **have** been taken from the same population.

If the calculated value falls within the range generated by the most extreme 5% of departures from the null hypothesis, the result is considered statistically significant. Most statistical packages give the value of the test statistic, together with the probability of that outcome. Randomisation and exact tests can also be used to compare two or more samples of ratio, interval, or ordinal data, and are described in this chapter.

18.2   A non-parametric comparison between one sample and an expected distribution

The Kolmogorov–Smirnov one-sample test can be used to compare the distribution of a single sample with an expected or known distribution. For example, if you were interested in examining whether the growth rate (measured by the weight gained) of pigs raised on organic farms during their first year of life was different to factory reared pigs, you might have data for 36 'organic' pigs but no data for 36 equivalent factory grown controls. In this case you would have to test the hypothesis that the distribution of the weight gained by 'organic' pigs during their first year is no different to the known (population) distribution of weight gained during this time by factory grown pigs.

Here is an example. Data for the increase in weight in kilograms for the 36 organically reared pigs during their first year are shown below:

10.1, 12.2, 18.6, 19.5, 13.6, 17.5, 14.0, 20.2, 11.7, 15.8, 18.4, 19.2, 11.8, 19.6, 12.4, 20.5, 12.9, 13.3, 13.7, 13.1, 12.8, 20.7, 20.9, 10.4, 11.4, 22.1, 21.7, 15.6, 19.3, 18.6, 16.2, 18.0, 23.0, 14.1, 12.5, 13.6

If you make a preliminary inspection of these data by drawing a histogram, you will find the distribution is bimodal and clearly not appropriate for analysis using a parametric test such as a one-sample t test. A non-parametric test is needed.

You can use a Kolmogorov–Smirnov one-sample test to compare this bimodal distribution with the known distribution of weight gained by factory reared pigs during their first year (which is also bimodal) and has been well established from such a large number of pigs over several decades that it can be assumed to be the distribution for the population.

First, you need to construct a table of frequencies that summarises these data, using the procedure for drawing a frequency histogram described in Section 3.3.2. Once you have decided on an interval number and width that

Table 18.1. A worked example of a Kolmogorov–Smirnov one-sample test. The numbers of pigs in each category are converted to proportions of the sample and then expressed as cumulative proportions, which are compared, by subtraction, with the known (expected) cumulative proportions for the population and expressed as the absolute difference. The greatest difference is identified. In this case it is 0.1217 (shown in bold in the far right-hand column), which is the value of D. If the probability of obtaining this or a more extreme value of D is less than 5% the sample is considered significantly different to the expected distribution

Category of weights	Observed numbers in each category	Observed proportion in each category	Observed cumulative proportions in each category	Expected cumulative proportions	Absolute difference (observed minus expected)
10–11.99	5	0.1389	0.1389	0.1045	0.0344
12–13.99	10	0.2778	0.4167	0.3943	0.0224
14–15.99	4	0.1111	0.5278	0.5623	0.0345
16–17.99	2	0.0556	0.5833	0.6236	0.0403
18–19.99	8	0.2222	0.8056	0.6839	**0.1217**
20–21.99	5	0.1389	0.9444	0.9325	0.0119
22–23.99	2	0.0556	1.0000	1.0000	0.0000
Total	36	1.0000			

will reveal the shape of the distribution (Section 3.3.2), you need to count the number of cases that fall within each interval (Table 18.1) and convert these to their proportions of the sample. Next, progressively add these proportions together to give the cumulative proportions. Here too, this procedure is the same as drawing a cumulative frequency graph (Section 3.3.3).

The cumulative proportions for the sample have to be compared with the cumulative proportions of the known distribution. To do this you calculate the absolute value of the difference between the observed and expected proportions in each interval, which will always be positive. The greatest difference is identified and called the D statistic.

If the observed and expected proportions in each interval are the same, the value of D will be zero. As the discrepancy between the observed and expected proportions increases, the value of D will increase and eventually exceed the critical value, which will depend on sample size. A worked example is given in Table 18.1. Statistical packages generate the cumulative frequency distributions, calculate D, and give the probability.

18.3   Non-parametric comparisons between two independent samples

18.3.1 The Mann–Whitney test

The Mann–Whitney test is used to compare two independent samples. First, the values are ranked **over both samples** as shown in Table 18.2, which gives data for the height of nine palm seedlings grown in two different soil types. The smallest value is given the rank of 1, the next largest the rank of 2 etc., so the largest will have the rank of $n_1 + n_2$ (which is the sum of the number of cases in both samples). For the data in Table 18.2, the largest possible rank is 9.

If two or more values are the same (that is, they are **tied**), each is given the average of the ranks assigned to that many values. For example, if the data in Table 18.2 contained two 4 cm high seedlings and these were the smallest, each would be given the average of ranks 1 and 2, which is 1.5.

If most of the seedlings grew taller in one soil type than the other, the ranks would differ between treatments. In contrast, if the seedlings grew to a similar height in both soil types, the ranks within each treatment would also be similar.

The ranks are summed separately for each sample (these are R_1 and R_2 in Table 18.2) and the two Mann–Whitney statistics U and U' calculated:

$$U = n_1 \times n_2 + \frac{n_1(n_1 + 1)}{2} - R_1 \tag{18.1}$$

and:

Table 18.2. The height, in centimetres, of palm seedlings germinated and grown for six weeks in clay soil and sandy soil. Ranks are shown in the two right-hand columns, together with the rank sums (R_1 and R_2) for each treatment

Height in clay soil	Height in sandy soil	Rank for clay soil	Rank for sandy soil
24	22	7	6
41	6	9	2
17	11	5	3
38	15	8	4
	4		1
$n_1 = 4$	$n_2 = 5$	$R_1 = 29$	$R_2 = 16$

$$U' = \quad n_1 \times n_2 + \frac{n_2(n_2 + 1)}{2} - R_2 \qquad (18.2)$$

where n_1 and n_2 are the size of each sample.

These formulae may appear complex, but are easily explained by separating them into three components as shown for U in equation (18.3).

$$U = \quad \underbrace{n_1 \times n_2}_{\text{component A}} \quad + \quad \underbrace{\frac{n_1(n_1 + 1)}{2}}_{\text{component B}} \quad - \quad \underbrace{R_1}_{\text{component C}} \qquad (18.3)$$

Component A will increase with the size of both samples. Component B will only increase as the size of sample 1 increases. In contrast, component C will be affected by the way the ranks are distributed between the two samples. A lot of low ranks in sample 1 will give a relatively small value of R_1 and *vice versa*. Therefore, since U is calculated by taking component C away from the sum of components A and B, it will be large compared with U' when sample 1 contains mainly low ranks. In contrast, if sample 1 contains mainly high ranks, the value of U will be small compared with U'. Finally, if both samples contain similar ranks, then neither U nor U' will be relatively large or small.

When both samples are from the same population, most values of U and U' will be similar, but differences between them will occur by chance and the most extreme 5% of discrepancies will give values of U or U' that will be equal to, or exceed, a critical value. For a two-tailed test, if **either** of the U statistics exceeds the critical value, then the probability that the samples are from the same population is less than 5%.

18.3.2 Randomisation tests for two independent samples

Another way of comparing two independent samples, without assuming they are from a normal distribution, is to use a randomisation test. These tests were first discussed in relation to samples of categorical data in Chapter 17.

If two independent samples are taken from the same population, then the values within each should differ only by chance. A randomisation test takes the combined set of ranks from both samples (a group of size $n_1 + n_2$), repeatedly samples it at random, and assigns the ranks to two groups of size n_1 and n_2.

The simulated sampling is iterated several thousand times and used to generate the **expected** distribution of U and U' from the data set and therefore identify the most extreme 5% of departures from the outcome expected under the null hypothesis. Finally, the U statistics for the actual outcome are compared with these distributions and, if the probability is less than 5%, it is statistically significant (Figure 18.1).

18.3.3 Exact tests for two independent samples

Data for two samples can also be analysed by tests that calculate the exact probability, and work in a very similar way to the Fisher Exact Probability Test described in Chapter 17.

An exact test for two independent samples calculates the probability of the actual difference (or values of statistics such as U and U') between the ranks of the samples, together with any more extreme differences from the outcome expected under the null hypothesis. This gives the one-tailed probability of the outcome.

Here is an example for two independent samples with three data in each. The values range from 1 to 6, and the total set of ways in which they can be distributed between two samples is shown in Table 18.3. I have deliberately made the values the same as their ranks, and used a simple comparison between the rank sums of the samples.

For this example there are only two combinations that will give the greatest difference between the rank sums. These are when the first sample contains the three lowest (1, 2, and 3) and the second the three highest (4, 5, and 6) ranks and vice versa, giving an absolute difference of nine. Less extreme differences can be obtained from several combinations and are therefore more likely (Table 18.3).

For example, you may wish to calculate the probability of the observed outcome and any more extreme departures from the one expected under the null hypothesis when one sample contains the ranks 1, 2, and 5 (and the other contains ranks 3, 4, and 6). The observed difference between the sums of the ranks is -5. You will find this outcome in the third line from the top of Table 18.3. There are two more extreme differences (-7 and -9) in the same direction (that is, with increasingly negative values) from the

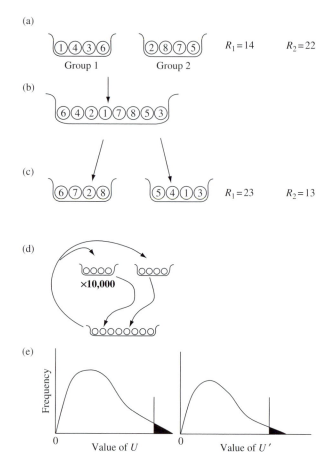

Figure 18.1 Illustration of a randomisation procedure that gives distributions of the two Mann-Whitney statistics U and U' from simulated sampling, which can be used to decide whether an observed outcome is statistically significant. (a) The actual outcome of the expriment. (b) The ranks from both groups are combined. (c) The combined set of ranks is resampled at random to give two more groups of size n_1 and n_2 and thereby generate two new values of R_1 and R_2. (d) Steps (b) and (c) are repeated several thousand times. Each time, two more values of R_1 and R_2 are generated. (e) The simulated sampling gives the distributions of U and U' for two samples taken at random from the same group. By chance there will often be differences between samples, and as they increase so will U or U'. The largest 5% of the values of U and U' are shown as the filled areas on the right of each graph. Finally, the U statistics from the actual outcome (a) are compared with these distributions. If the probability of getting either U or U' is less than 5% (i.e. either statistic falls within the filled area), the null hypothesis that the samples in (a) are from the same population is rejected.

Table 18.3. The set of ways in which six ranks can be distributed between two samples of three. Note that the most extreme differences (of -9 and 9) between the sums of the ranks of two samples can only be obtained when one contains ranks 1, 2, and 3 and the other 4, 5, and 6, so these outcomes have a relatively low probability compared with less extreme differences (e.g. 1 and -1), which can be obtained in several different ways

Sample 1			Rank sums and their differences	Sample 2		
(a)	(b)	(c)		(c)	(b)	(a)
1						4
2			$R_1 = 6\ R_1 - R_2 = -9\ R_2 = 15$			5
3						6
1						3
2			$R_1 = 7\ R_1 - R_2 = -7\ R_2 = 14$			5
4						6
1	1				2	3
2	3		$R_1 = 8\ R_1 - R_2 = -5\ R_2 = 13$		5	4
5	4				6	6
2	1	1		3	2	1
3	3	2	$R_1 = 9\ R_1 - R_2 = -3\ R_2 = 12$	4	4	5
4	5	6		5	6	6
2	1	1		2	2	1
3	3	4	$R_1 = 10\ R_1 - R_2 = -1\ R_2 = 11$	3	4	4
5	6	5		6	5	6
1	2	2		1	1	2
4	4	3	$R_1 = 11\ R_1 - R_2 = 1\ R_2 = 10$	2	3	3
6	5	6		5	6	5
1	2	3		1	1	2
5	4	4	$R_1 = 12\ R_1 - R_2 = 3\ R_2 = 9$	2	3	3
6	6	5		6	5	4
3	2			1	1	
4	5		$R_1 = 13\ R_1 - R_2 = 5\ R_2 = 8$	3	2	
6	6			4	5	
3						1
5			$R_1 = 14\ R_1 - R_2 = 7\ R_2 = 7$			2
6						4
4						1
5			$R_1 = 15\ R_1 - R_2 = 9\ R_2 = 6$			2
6						3

outcome expected under the null hypothesis. The probability of each outcome is calculated directly from sampling a set of six values without replacement (e.g. the chance of rank 1 is 1/6, but the chance of then selecting rank 2 is 1/5 etc.). Once calculated, these probabilities are summed and thus give the one-tailed probability of the observed outcome and any more extreme departures from the null hypothesis. The probability is one-tailed, because differences in the same absolute size between the samples (i.e. the last three lines showing differences of 5, 7, and 9) in Table 18.3 have been ignored, and has to be doubled to get the two-tailed probability.

18.3.4 Recommended non-parametric tests for two independent samples

If you have a statistical package that includes an exact or randomisation test for two independent samples, either of these is recommended in preference to the Mann–Whitney test.

18.4   Non-parametric comparisons among more than two independent samples

The most frequently used non-parametric test for more than two independent samples is the Kruskal–Wallis test. It is also called the Kruskal–Wallis single factor analysis of variance by ranks, but this is misleading because it does not use analysis of variance to compare samples. Instead, the Kruskal–Wallis test is an extension of the Mann–Whitney test that can be applied to three or more samples.

18.4.1 The Kruskal–Wallis test

For a Kruskal–Wallis test the data are ranked in the same way as for a Mann–Whitney test, starting by assigning the lowest rank to the smallest value. Here is an example for the number of sandfly bites on the arms of 16 college students who spent three hours without insect repellent while on a class field trip to a Florida mangrove swamp (Table 18.4). The students were classified into three groups according to their natural hair colour and

Table 18.4. The number of sandfly bites on both arms of 16 students, who did not wear insect repellent, after spending three hours in a Florida mangrove swamp. Five had black hair, six had brown hair, and five were blonde. The totals are the rank sums within each group

	Number of sandfly bites			Number of sandfly bites ranked from the least to most	
Black hair	Brown hair	Blonde hair	Black hair	Brown Hair	Blonde hair
25	31	22	9	13	8
14	20	4	4	7	1
35	29	11	14	11	3
41	15	18	16	5	6
28	40	8	10	15	2
	30			12	
		Total	$R_1 = 53$	$R_2 = 63$	$R_3 = 20$

the null hypothesis was, 'There is no difference in the number of sandfly bites on the arms of people with different hair colour.'

It is clear that a marked difference in the number of sandfly bites among groups will also result in a difference in the ranks and rank sums.

The rank sums for each group are used in the following formula for the Kruskal–Wallis statistic H:

$$H = \frac{12}{N(N+1)} \sum_{i=1}^{k} R_i^2 - 3(N+1) \tag{18.4}$$

where N is the **total** sample size and k is the number of groups or samples. Although this formula looks complex, it is straightforward when considered as three components:

$$H = \underbrace{\frac{12}{N(N+1)}}_{\text{component A}} \times \underbrace{\sum_{i=1}^{k} R_i^2}_{\text{component B}} - \underbrace{3(N+1)}_{\text{component C}} \tag{18.5}$$

Components A and C will increase as sample size increases. Component B is the sum of all the squared rank totals. If all R_i values are relatively similar,

Box 18.1 The effect of an unequal allocation of ranks on the total of the squared rank sums

This example uses three groups with two values in each. Only the ranks of the values are shown. First, the rank sums are identical among groups.

Group A	Group B	Group C
1	2	3
6	5	4
$R_1 = 7$	$R_2 = 7$	$R_3 = 7$

$$\sum_{i=1}^{k} R_i^2 = 3 \times 49 = 147$$

Second, the rank sums are different among groups and this gives a larger sum of the squared rank sums.

Group A	Group B	Group C
1	3	5
2	4	6
$R_1 = 3$	$R_2 = 7$	$R_3 = 11$

$$\sum_{i=1}^{k} R_i^2 = 3^2 + 7^2 + 11^2 = 179$$

then component B (and therefore H) will be smaller, than when some are large and others small, because of the effect of squaring relatively large numbers (Box 18.1).

The distribution of H for samples taken at random from the same population has been established and used to identify the 5% most extreme departures from the null hypothesis of no difference. For large samples, or where the number of groups or treatments is more than five, the value of H

is a close approximation to the chi-square statistic with $(k-1)$ degrees of freedom, and many statistical packages only give this statistic (and its probability) for the result of a Kruskal–Wallis test.

18.4.2 Exact tests and randomisation tests for three or more independent samples

Randomisation and exact tests on the ranks of three or more independent samples are extensions of the methods described for two independent samples in Section 18.3 and it is not necessary to explain these further.

18.4.3 A-posteriori comparisons after a non-parametric test

A non-parametric comparison can detect a significant difference among three or more groups, but it cannot show **which** groups appear to be from the same, or different, populations. This problem was discussed in Chapter 9 in relation to a single factor parametric ANOVA. If the effect of the variable you are examining is considered fixed, you need to use non-parametric a-posteriori tests to compare among groups. These are described in more advanced texts (e.g. Sprent, 1993).

18.4.4 Rank transformation followed by one factor ANOVA

Another way of analysing data that are grossly non-normal is to run a parametric single factor ANOVA on the ranks. This is not a true non-parametric test, but has the advantage of easy a-posteriori comparisons when an effect is fixed and the initial analysis shows a significant difference among samples. It is as powerful as applying a Kruskal–Wallis test.

18.4.5 Recommended non-parametric tests for three or more independent samples

Most statistical packages include the Kruskal–Wallis test, which is up to 95% as powerful as the equivalent parametric single factor ANOVA described in Chapter 9. If you have a package that includes an exact test or randomisation test, these are recommended in preference to the

Kruskal–Wallis test. Several texts recommend using a parametric ANOVA after rank transformation but it is important to note that this is not a true non-parametric comparison.

18.5 Non-parametric comparisons of two related samples

Related samples were first discussed in Chapter 7. Some examples are when a variable is measured twice (and usually under different conditions) on the same experimental unit, or when the experimental units within one sample or treatment are somehow related to those in a second (e.g. an experiment with two treatments, where a pair of rats is taken from each of several litters and one in each pair assigned to different treatments). There are several non-parametric tests for determining the probability that two related samples have been taken from the same population. These include the Wilcoxon paired-sample test, as well as randomisation and exact tests for this statistic.

18.5.1 The Wilcoxon paired-sample test

The Wilcoxon paired-sample test is the non-parametric equivalent of the paired sample *t* test. The following example is for two samples taken from each of ten experimental units. In humans the trachea branches into two bronchi, which lead to different lungs. The bronchus leading to the right lung is wider, shorter, and angled more closely to the vertical than the one leading to the left lung. Not surprisingly, it has been found that inhaled objects are more likely to lodge in the right bronchus, so a pathologist hypothesised the right lung may also receive a greater proportion of inhaled airborne particles such as smoke, and therefore be more prone to damage. To test this, the pathologist counted the number of lesions found during post mortem examination of the left and right lungs of ten males who had died of natural causes. The data are in Table 18.5.

For the Wilcoxon test the difference between each pair of related samples is first calculated. This is also expressed as the absolute difference and these values ranked (Table 18.5). Finally, the ranks associated with negative and

Table 18.5. Data for the number of separate lesions found during post mortem examination of the left and right lungs of ten males who died from natural causes. For a Wilcoxon test the difference between each pair of related data is calculated (d), expressed as the absolute difference (e), and these absolute values ranked (f). The ranks associated with positive differences (h) and negative differences (i) are separately summed to give the statistics $T+$ and $T-$

(a) Specimen number	(b) Right lung	(c) Left lung	(d) Difference (right–left)	(e) Absolute difference	(f) Rank of the absolute differences	(g) Sign of the difference	(h) Ranks associated with positive differences	(i) Ranks associated with negative differences
1	19	15	4	4	2	+	2	
2	24	14	10	10	6	+	6	
3	16	22	−6	6	4	−		4
4	28	28	0	0	1	+	1	
5	19	11	8	8	5	+	5	
6	26	9	17	17	8	+	8	
7	16	38	−22	22	10	−		10
8	27	42	−15	15	7	−		7
9	18	13	5	5	3	+	3	
10	18	37	−19	19	9	−		9
						Totals	$T+=25$	$T-=30$

positive differences are summed separately to give the Wilcoxon statistics $T+$ and $T-$. For the data in Table 18.4, the ranks of the positive differences sum to 25 (cases 1, 2, 4, 5, 6, and 9), while the ranks of the negative differences sum to 30 (cases 3, 7, 8, and 10).

Under the null hypothesis of no effect of bronchial structure on the number of lesions in each lung, any difference between each pair of related samples (and therefore $T+$ and $T-$) would only be expected by chance. If, however, there were an effect of bronchial structure, it would contribute to differences between these two statistics.

The values of $T+$ and $T-$ can be compared with their expected distributions by taking related samples at random from a population. For a two-tailed test the null hypothesis is rejected if **either** $T+$ or $T-$ is **less** than a critical value, but for a one-tailed test the null hypothesis is only rejected if the appropriate T statistic is less than a critical value. For example, if it were hypothesised there were more lesions in the right lung than the left, a reduction in the number of negative ranks would be expected, so the null hypothesis would only be rejected if $T-$ were less than the critical value.

For large samples the distributions of both T statistics approximate the normal curve, so statistical packages often give the value of the Z statistic and probability for the result of the Wilcoxon test.

18.5.2 Exact tests and randomisation tests for two related samples

The procedures for randomisation and exact tests on the ranks of two related samples are conceptually similar to the analyses for two independent samples described in Section 18.3 and it is not necessary to explain them any further.

18.6   Non-parametric comparisons among three or more related samples

Tests for three or more related samples include the Friedman test, together with randomisation and exact tests for this statistic.

Table 18.6. The increase in weight, in kilograms, for piglets from six litters assigned to three different treatments. Piglets in the control treatment were offered unlimited food, while those in treatments A and B were offered unlimited food plus antibiotic A and B respectively

Litter	Control	Antibiotic A	Antibiotic B	Rank of control	Rank of A	Rank of B
1	2.5	2.7	2.1	2	3	1
2	1.8	1.9	2.0	1	2	3
3	4.4	4.7	4.1	2	3	1
4	2.4	2.6	2.3	2	3	1
5	5.1	5.3	5.2	1	3	2
6	1.7	1.9	1.6	2	3	1
			Totals	$R_1 = 10$	$R_2 = 17$	$R_3 = 9$

18.6.1 The Friedman test

The Friedman test is often called the Friedman two way (or two factor) analysis of variance by ranks, but this is misleading because it is not equivalent to the two factor ANOVA discussed in Chapter 11. The Friedman test cannot detect interaction and only examines differences among the levels of one factor, so is really analogous to the two factor ANOVA without replication applied to the randomised block experimental design described in Chapter 13.

For a Friedman test the data are first transformed to ranks. Table 18.6 gives the results of an experiment designed to compare the effects of two different antibiotics on the growth of pigs. Considerable differences in growth can occur among pigs from different litters, so each treatment was assigned one piglet from each of six litters, in a randomised block design with three treatments and six blocks. Piglets in the control treatment were offered unlimited food, while those in the other two treatments were offered unlimited food laced with either antibiotic A or antibiotic B. Data for the increase in weight of each piglet during the next two months are in Table 18.6.

First, ranks are assigned **within each block** and therefore within each row of Table 18.5. The lowest value in each row is given the rank of '1', the next highest '2' etc, and the highest rank cannot exceed the number of treatments.

If the treatments are from the same population, the range of ranks (and the rank sums) for each should be similar, with any variation due to chance. If, however, there is any effect of either treatment, the ranks and their sums will also differ. For the example in Table 18.6, antibiotic treatment A contains all but one of the highest ranks, while treatment B contains all but two of the lowest.

Second, the total of the squared rank sums is calculated. The size of this total will depend on the relative size of the rank sums (Box 18.1) with a set of similar ones giving a smaller total than a set of dissimilar ones.

Finally the following formula is used to calculate the Friedman statistic χ_r^2:

$$\chi_r^2 = \frac{12}{ba(a+1)} \sum_{i=1}^{a} R_i^2 - 3b(a+1) \tag{18.6}$$

where a is the number of treatments or groups and b is the number of blocks. This appears complex, but can be split into three components as shown in equation (18.7) below. The Friedman statistic is obtained by multiplying components A and B together and then subtracting component C.

$$\chi_r^2 = \underbrace{\frac{12}{ba(a+1)}}_{\text{component A}} \times \underbrace{\sum_{i=1}^{a} tR_i^2}_{\text{component B}} - \underbrace{3b(a+1)}_{\text{component C}} \tag{18.7}$$

Components A and C will increase as sample sizes and the number of samples increase. If the rank sums are very similar among treatments, component B will be relatively small, so the value of the Friedman statistic will also be small. As the differences among the rank sums increase, component B will increase, thus giving a larger value of the Friedman statistic. Once this exceeds the critical value above which less than 5% of the most extreme departures from the null hypothesis occur when samples are taken from the same population, the outcome is considered statistically significant.

This analysis can be up to 95% as powerful as the equivalent two way ANOVA without replication for randomised blocks.

18.6.2 Exact tests and randomisation tests for three or more related samples

The procedures for randomisation and exact tests on the ranks of three or more related samples are extensions of the methods for two independent samples and do not need to be explained any further.

18.6.3 A-posteriori comparisons for three or more related samples

If the Friedman test shows a significant difference among treatments and the effect is considered fixed, you are likely to want to know which treatments are significantly different (see 18.4.3). A-posteriori testing can be done and instructions are given in more advanced texts, such as Zar (1999).

18.7   Analysing ratio, interval, or ordinal data that show gross differences in variance among treatments and cannot be satisfactorily transformed

Some data show gross differences in variance among treatments that **cannot** be improved by transformation and are therefore unsuitable for parametric or non-parametric analysis. A peridontologist was asked to assess the effects of a dental hygiene program upon the incidence of caries among 14–19 year old adolescent males. Thirty males aged 14 years were chosen at random within a large high school. Fifteen were assigned at random to a 'hygiene' group and regularly encouraged to eat only three meals a day, carefully clean and floss their teeth after every meal, and reduce their consumption of carbonated sugary drinks, while the 15 students in the other group received no encouragement about dental hygiene. Members of both groups had regular dental examinations. The number of new cases of dental caries recorded during the next five years for each student are given in Table 18.7.

It is clear there are gross differences in variance among the treatments that cannot be remedied by transformation. The variance of the control group is 15.11, compared with 0.12 in the 'hygiene' group and the large

Table 18.7. The number of cases of new dental caries occurring in two groups of males between the ages of 14 and 19 years. The members of the 'hygiene' group were encouraged to undertake a rigorous dental hygiene program, while those in the control received no encouragement about dental hygiene

Control	Hygiene
4	0
7	0
4	0
10	0
2	0
7	0
1	0
9	1
3	0
9	0
12	1
7	0
5	0
4	0
15	0

Table 18.8. Transformation of the ratio data in Table 18.6 to a nominal scale showing the number of new caries within two mutually exclusive categories

	Control	Hygiene
Number without new caries	0	13
Number with new caries	15	2

number of zeros makes it impossible to satisfactorily reduce this heteroscedasticity.

One solution is to transform the data to a nominal scale and reclassify both samples into two mutually exclusive categories of 'no new caries' and 'new caries' (Table 18.8), which can be compared using a test for two independent samples of categorical data (Chapter 17).

18.8 Non-parametric correlation analysis

Correlation analysis was introduced in Chapter 14 as an exploratory technique used to examine whether two variables are related or **vary together**. Importantly, there is no expectation that the numerical value of one variable can be predicted from the other, nor is it necessary that either variable is determined by the other.

The parametric test for correlation gives a statistic that varies between +1.00 and −1.00, with both of these extremes indicating a perfect positive and negative straight line relationship respectively, while values around zero show no relationship. Although parametric correlation analysis is powerful, it can only detect linear relationships and also assumes that both the X and Y variables are normally distributed. When normality of both variables cannot be assumed, or the relationship between the two variables does not appear to be linear and cannot be remedied by transformation, it is not appropriate to use a parametric test for correlation.

The most commonly used non-parametric test for correlation is Spearman's rank correlation.

18.8.1 Spearman's rank correlation

This test is extremely straightforward. The two variables are ranked separately, from lowest to highest, and the (parametric) Pearson correlation coefficient calculated for the ranked values. This gives a statistic called Spearman's rho, which for a population is symbolised by ρ_s and by r_s for a sample.

Spearman's r_s and Pearson's r will not always be the same for the same set of data. For Pearson's r the correlation coefficients of 1.00 or −1.00 were only obtained when there was a perfect positive or negative straight-line relationship between the two variables. In contrast, Spearman's r_s will give a value of 1.00 or −1.00 whenever the ranks for the two variables are in perfect agreement or disagreement, which occurs in more cases than a straight-line relationship (Figure 18.2).

The probability of the value of r_s can be obtained by comparing it with the expected distribution of this statistic and most statistical packages will give r_s together with its probability.

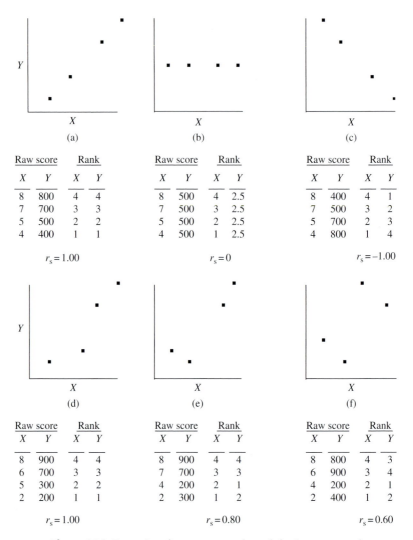

Figure 18.2 Examples of raw scores, ranks and the Spearman rank correlation coefficient for data with (a) A perfect positive relationship (all points lie along a straight line). (b) No relationship. (c) A perfect negative relationship (all points lie along a straight line). (d) A positive relationship which is not a straight line but all pairs of bivariate data have the same ranks. (e) A positive relationship with only half the pairs of bivariate data having equal ranks. (f) A positive relationship with no pairs of bivariate data having equal ranks. Note that the value of r_s is 1.00 for case (d) even though the raw data do not show a straight line relationship.

18.9   Other non-parametric tests

This chapter is only an introduction to some non-parametric tests for two or more samples of independent and related data. Other non-parametric tests are described in more specialised but nevertheless extremely well-explained texts, such as Siegel and Castallan (1988).

19 | Choosing a test

19.1   Introduction

Statisticians and life scientists who teach statistics are often visited in their offices by a researcher or student they may have never met before, who is clutching a dauntingly thick pile of paper and perhaps a couple of CDs with labels like 'Experiment 1' or 'Trial 2'. The visitor sits down, drops everything heavily on the desk, and says, 'Here are my results. What stats do I need?'

This is not a good thing to do. First, the person whose advice you are seeking may not have the time to work out exactly how you have done the experiment, so they may give you bad advice. Second, the answer can be a very nasty surprise like, 'There are problems with your experimental design'.

The decision about the appropriate statistical analysis needs to be made by considering the hypothesis being tested, the experimental design, and the type of data. It can save a lot of time, trouble, and disappointment if you think about possible ways of analysing the data **at the time the experiment is designed**, rather than only after the data have been collected.

The following tables are a guide to choosing an appropriate test. You need to start at Table 19.1, which initially gives three columns that are mutually exclusive choices. Once you have decided among these, work downwards within the column you have chosen. There may be more choices and here you also need to select the appropriate column and continue downwards. Eventually you will be referred to another table with more choices that lead to suggested tests.

Table 19.1. The first step in deciding which test to use is to ask if the hypothesis is about: (a) whether one sample is from population with known or expected statistics, (b) whether two or more samples are from the same population, or (c) whether two variables are related

Is the hypothesis being tested by examining whether:		
One sample is from a population with known statistics?	Two or more samples are from the same population?	Two variables are related?

Two or more samples are from the same population?

Are the data measured on a **ratio, interval, or ordinal** scale and give the value of a variable for each experimental unit? (For example, data for the heart rate of athletes in two or more groups or treatments?)

Two variables are related?

Data must be **bivariate** measured on a **ratio, interval, or ordinal scale** and can be displayed as a two dimensional scatter plot

Case	X	Y
1	2	7
2	4	11
3	6	13
4	8	15
5	10	18
6	12	19
7	14	22
8	16	23

Go to Table 19.8

One sample is from a population with known statistics?

The data may be **ratio, interval, or ordinal** scale or **nominal** scale (example (a) below) or (example (b) below)

Are the data measured on a **nominal** scale as two or more mutually exclusive categories in independent samples (example (a) below) or two or more related samples (example (b) below)?

Are the samples independent?

Case	Sample 1	Sample 2	Sample 3
1	X		
2	X		
3		X	
4		X	
5			X
6			X

Are the data grossly non-normal?

Go to Table 19.4

Can you assume the data are normally distributed?

Go to Table 19.5

Are the samples related?

Case	Sample 1	Sample 2	Sample 3
1	X	X	X
2	X	X	X
3	X	X	X
4	X	X	X
5	X	X	X
6	X	X	X

Can you assume the data are normally distributed?

Got to Table 19.6

Are the data grossly non-normal?

Go to Table 19.7

(a) The height in cm for a sample of five individuals

Case	Height
1	165
2	150
3	159
4	145
5	170

(b) The number of males and females in a sample of 200:

Female	Male
107	93

Go to Table 19.2

(a) The number of male and female whelks in baited traps at several sites:

	Site 1	Site 2	Site 3
Female	32	21	36
Male	14	23	17

(b) Responses of the same individual before and after feeding:

Case	Response before	Response after
1	Yes	No
2	Yes	No
3	No	No
4	Yes	No
5	No	No

Go to Table 19.3

Table 19.2. Tests for one sample

To test whether one sample is from a population with known statistics		
Are the data measured on a **nominal** scale as the frequencies in two or more mutually exclusive categories? (For example, the numbers of male and female whelks in a baited trap for comparison with an expected sex ratio of 1:1.) 	Male	Female
---	---
54	56 | **Non-parametric goodness of fit test** (Chapter 17)	Are the data measured on a **ratio, interval, or ordinal** scale? (For example, data for the height of several individuals).	
	Is the sample from a population that appears normal, or not grossly non-normal? Y X **Z test** if population mean and variance are known (Chapter 7) but **single sample *t* test** if there is only an expected value for the population mean (Chapter 7)	Is the sample from a population that is grossly non-normal (e.g. bimodal?) Y X **Kolmogorov–Smirnov one-sample test** (Chapter 18)

Table 19.3. Tests for two or more samples of nominal scale data

To test whether two or more samples of nominal scale data are from the same population

Are the samples independent?

Can the data be cast as a 2 × 2 table?

	Sample 1	Sample 2
Alive	12	33
Dead	42	27

A Fisher Exact test or a chi-square test for a 2 × 2 contingency table (Chapter 17)

Caution: For small sample sizes a Fisher Exact Test is more accurate

Can the data be cast as a $k \times k$ table?

	Sample 1	Sample 2	Sample 3
Red	23	14	24
Yellow	12	19	14
Brown	4	5	2

A chi-square test, exact test or randomisation test for a $k \times k$ contingency table (Chapter 17)

Caution: Exact tests are more accurate when sample sizes are small

Are the samples related?

Are there two samples?

Case	Condition 1	Condition 2
1	Yes	No
2	Yes	No
3	No	No
4	Yes	Yes
5	No	No
6	Yes	No

A McNemar test for the significance of changes or an exact or randomisation test (Chapter 17)

Are there more than two samples?

Case	Condition 1	Condition 2	Condition 3
1	Yes	No	No
2	Yes	No	Yes
3	No	No	No
4	Yes	Yes	Yes
5	No	No	Yes
6	Yes	No	No

A Cochran Q test or an exact or randomisation test (Chapter 17)

Table 19.4. Tests for two or more independent samples of normally distributed ratio, interval, or ordinal scale data

To test whether two or more independent samples of normally distributed ratio, interval, or ordinal scale data are from the same population

Are the data replicates for two or more levels of a single factor (e.g. growth at three different temperatures)?

20°C	30°C	40°C
6	13	28
3	17	26
1	20	23
4	16	26

	Two samples	Three or more samples
Sample variances similar	Independent sample *t* test (Chapter 7) or single factor ANOVA (Chapter 9)	Single factor ANOVA (Chapter 9)
Sample variances grossly dissimilar	Independent sample *t* test (Chapter 7), which does not assume equal variances.	Transform and recheck. If similar, use single factor ANOVA (Chapter 9). If not, analyse with caution because of the increased risk of Type 1 error (Chapter 12)

Are the data an orthogonal design for two or more levels of two factors (e.g. growth in relation to temperature and light intensity)?

20°C		30°C		40°C	
High light	Low light	High light	Low light	High light	Low light
6	1	13	3	28	5
3	3	17	5	26	7
1	2	20	2	23	3
4	1	16	5	26	4

Data are replicated within each combination of treatments

Variances are similar among treatment combinations	**Two factor ANOVA** (Chapter 11)
Variances are grossly dissimilar among treatment combinations	**Transform** and recheck variances. If similar, use **two factor ANOVA** (Chapter 11). Otherwise, use ANOVA, but be aware of the increased risk of Type 1 error (Chapter 12)

Data are not replicated.

Two factor ANOVA without replication (Chapter 13).

Are the data an orthogonal design for two or more levels of three or more factors (e.g. growth in relation to temperature, light intensity, and humidity)?

Three factor or higher ANOVA subject to the cautions and conditions for two factor ANOVA in the columns to the left of this one

Are the data a nested design where one or more factors are nested within the levels of another? (For example, the effect of temperature on growth, with two growth chambers nested within each temperature)

20°C		30°C		40°C	
Chamber A	B	Chamber C	D	Chamber E	F
6	5	13	15	28	34
3	6	17	19	26	19
2	1	20	13	23	26
1	1	16	17	26	28

Nested ANOVA (Chapter 13), subject to the cautions about inequality of variances noted in the columns for single factor and two factor ANOVA to the left of this one

Table 19.5. Tests for two or more independent samples of ratio, interval, or ordinal scale data that are not normally distributed

To test whether two or more independent samples of ratio, interval, or ordinal scale data, that are grossly non-normal, are from the same population				
Are the data for two levels or samples of one factor (e.g. growth at two different temperatures)?		Are the data for three or more levels or samples of one factor (e.g. growth at three different temperatures)?		
20°C	30°C	20°C	30°C	40°C
6	13	6	13	28
3	17	3	17	26
1	20	1	20	23
4	16	4	16	26
Sample distributions similar	Sample distributions grossly different	Sample distributions similar		Sample distributions grossly different
Mann–Whitney U test, randomisation test or exact test (Chapter 18)	Transform to a nominal scale and analyse as categorical data (Chapter 18)	Kruskal–Wallis test, randomisation test, or exact test (Chapter 18)		Transform to a nominal scale and analyse as categorical data (Chapter 18)

Table 19.6. Tests for two or more related samples of normally distributed ratio, interval, or ordinal scale data

To test whether two or more related samples of normally distributed data are from the same population						
Two related samples			**Three or more related samples**			
Case	Sample 1	Sample 2	Case	Sample 1	Sample 2	Sample 3
1	12	15	1	12	15	23
2	16	12	2	16	12	18
3	21	17	3	21	17	26
4	18	10	4	18	10	21
5	19	14	5	19	14	29
6	12	18	6	12	18	24
Paired sample *t* test (Chapter 7) **or two factor ANOVA without replication** (Chapter 13)			**Two factor ANOVA without replication** (Chapter 13)			

Table 19.7. Tests for two or more related samples of ratio, interval, or ordinal scale data that are not normally distributed

	To test whether two or more related samples of data, that are grossly non-normal, are from the same population						
	Two related samples			Three or more related samples			
Case	Sample 1	Sample 2		Case	Sample 1	Sample 2	Sample 3
1	12	15		1	12	15	23
2	16	12		2	16	12	18
3	21	17		3	21	17	26
4	18	10		4	18	10	21
5	19	14		5	19	14	29
6	12	18		6	12	18	24
Wilcoxon paired-sample test, randomisation test or exact test (Chapter 18).				Friedman test, randomisation test or exact test (Chapter 18).			

Table 19.8. Tests for whether two variables are related

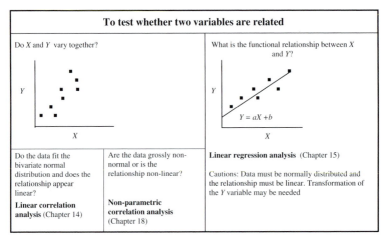

To test whether two variables are related		
Do X and Y vary together?		What is the functional relationship between X and Y?
Do the data fit the bivariate normal distribution and does the relationship appear linear?	Are the data grossly non-normal or is the relationship non-linear?	**Linear regression analysis** (Chapter 15)
Linear correlation analysis (Chapter 14)	**Non-parametric correlation analysis** (Chapter 18)	Cautions: Data must be normally distributed and the relationship must be linear. Transformation of the Y variable may be needed

20 | Doing science responsibly and ethically

20.1 Introduction

By now you are likely to have a very clear idea about how science is done. Science is the process of rational enquiry, which seeks explanations for natural phenomena. Scientific method was discussed in a very prescriptive way in Chapter 2 as the proposal of an hypothesis from which predictions are made and tested by doing experiments. Depending on the results, which may have to be analysed statistically, the decision is made to either retain or reject the hypothesis. This process of **knowledge by disproof** advances our understanding of the natural world and seems impartial and hard to fault.

Unfortunately, this is not necessarily the case, because **science is done by human beings who sometimes do not behave responsibly or ethically.** For example, some scientists fail to give credit to those who have helped propose a new hypothesis. Others make up, change, or delete results so their hypothesis is not rejected, omit details to prevent the detection of poor experimental design and deal unfairly with the work of others. Most scientists are not taught about responsible behaviour and are supposed to learn a code of conduct by example. Considering the number of cases of scientific irresponsibility that have been exposed, this does not seem to be a very good strategy. This chapter is about the importance of behaving responsibly and ethically when doing science.

20.2 Dealing fairly with other people's work

20.2.1 Plagiarism

Plagiarism is the theft and use of techniques, data, words, or ideas without appropriate acknowledgement. If you are using an experimental technique or procedure devised by someone else, or data owned by another person, you must acknowledge this. If you have been reading another person's work, it is easy to inadvertently use some of their phrases, but plagiarism is the repeated and excessive use of text without acknowledgement. Once your work is published any detected plagiarism can affect your credibility and your career.

20.2.2 Acknowledging previous work

Previous studies can be extremely valuable since they may add weight to an hypothesis and even suggest other hypotheses to test. There is a surprising tendency for scientists to fail to acknowledge previous published work by others in the same area, sometimes to the extent that experiments done two or three decades ago are repeated and presented as new findings. This can be an honest mistake in that the researcher is unaware of previous work, but the availability of electronic databases has made it far easier to search the scientific literature than it used to be. When you submit your work to a scientific journal for publication it can be embarrassing to be told that something similar has been done before. Even if a reviewer or editor of a journal does not notice, others may and are likely to say so in print.

20.2.3 Fair dealing

Some researchers cite the work done by others in the same field but downplay or even distort it. Although it appears that previous work in the field has been acknowledged, since the publication is listed in the references at the end of the paper or report, the researcher has nevertheless been somewhat dishonest. I have found this in about 5% of the papers I have reviewed, but it may be more common since it is quite hard to detect unless you are very familiar with the work. Often the problem seems to arise because the writer has only read the abstract of a paper, which can be misleading. It is important to carefully read and critically evaluate previous work in your field, because it will improve the quality of your own research.

20.2.4 Acknowledging the input of others

Often hypotheses may arise from discussions with colleagues or with your supervisor. This is an accepted aspect of how science is done. If, however, the discussion has been relatively one sided in that someone has suggested a useful and novel hypothesis to you, then you should seriously think about acknowledgement. One of my colleagues once said bitterly, 'My suggestions become someone else's original thoughts in a matter of seconds.' Acknowledgement can be a mention (in a section headed 'Acknowledgements') at the end of a report or paper, or you may even include the person as an author. It is not surprising that disputes often arise between supervisors and their postgraduate students about authorship of papers. Some supervisors argue that they have facilitated all of the student's work by being the supervisor and therefore expect their name to be included on all papers from the research. Others recognise the importance of the student having some single-authored papers and do not insist on this. The decision depends on the amount and type of input and rests with the principal author of the paper, but it is often helpful to clarify the matter of authorship and acknowledgement with your supervisor(s) at the start of a postgraduate program or new job.

20.3   Doing the experiment

20.3.1   Approval

You are likely to need prior permission or approval to do some types of research, or to work in a national park or reserve. Research on endangered species is very likely to need a permit (or permits) and you will have to give a good reason for doing the work, including its likely advantages and disadvantages. In many countries there are severe penalties for breaches of permits or doing research without one.

20.3.2   Ethics

Ethics are moral judgements where you have to decide if something is right or wrong, so different scientists can have different ethical views. Ethical issues include honesty and fair dealing, but they also extend to whether experimental procedures can be justified – for example procedures which kill, mutilate, or are thought to cause pain or suffering to animals. Some scientists think it is right to test cosmetic products on animals, because it will reduce the likelihood of harming or causing pain to humans, while others think it is wrong, because it may cause pain and suffering to the animals. Both groups would probably find it odd if someone said it was unethical to do experiments on insects or plants. Importantly, however, none of these three views can be considered the best or most appropriate, because ethical standards are not absolute. Provided a person honestly believes, for any reason, that it is right to do what they are doing, they are behaving ethically (Singer, 1992) and it is up to you to decide what is right. The remainder of this section is about the ethical conduct of research, rather than whether a research topic or procedure is considered ethical.

Research on vertebrates, which appear to feel pain, is likely to require approval by an animal ethics committee in the organisation where you are working. The committee will consider the likely advantages and disadvantages of the research, the number of animals used, possible alternative procedures, and the likelihood the animals will experience pain and suffering, and your research proposal may not necessarily be approved. Taking a wider view, research on any living organism has the potential to affect that species and others, so all life scientists should think carefully about their experimental procedures and should try to minimise disturbance, deaths, and possible suffering.

Most research organisations also have strict ethical guidelines on using humans in experiments. Any procedures need to be considered carefully in terms of the benefits, disadvantages, possible pain and suffering, together with issues of maintaining privacy and confidentiality, before being submitted to the human ethics committee for approval. Once again, the committee may not approve the research. There are usually strict reporting requirements and severe penalties for breaches of the procedure specified by the permit.

20.4   Evaluating and reporting results

Once you have the results of an experiment you need to analyse and discuss them in terms of rejection or retention of your hypothesis. Unfortunately some scientists have been known to change the results of experiments to make them consistent with their hypothesis, which is grossly dishonest. I suspect it is more common than reported and may even be fostered by assessment procedures in universities and colleges, where marks are given for the correct outcomes of practical experiments.

I once asked an undergraduate statistics class how many people had ever altered their data to fit the expectations of their biology practical assignments and got a lot of very guilty looks. I know two researchers who were dishonest. The first had a regression line that was not statistically significant, so they changed the data until it was. The second made up entire sets of data for sampling that had never been done. Both were found out and neither is still doing science.

It has been suggested that part of the problem stems from people becoming attached to their hypotheses and believing they are true, which goes completely against science proceeding by disproof! Some researchers are quite downcast when results are inconsistent with their hypothesis, but you need to be impartial about the results of any experiment and remember that a negative result is just as important as a positive one, because our understanding of the natural world has progressed in both cases.

Another cause of dishonesty is that scientists are often under extraordinary pressure to provide evidence for a particular hypothesis. There are often career rewards for finding solutions to problems or suggesting new models of natural processes. Competition among scientists for jobs, promotion, and recognition is intense and can also foster dishonesty.

The problem with scientific dishonesty is that the person has not reported what is really occurring. Science aims to describe the real world, so, if you fail to reject an hypothesis when a result suggests you should, you will report a false and misleading view of the process under investigation. Future hypotheses and research are likely to produce results inconsistent with your findings. There have been some spectacular cases where scientific dishonesty has been revealed, which has only served to undermine the credibility of the scientific process.

20.4.1 Pressure from peers or superiors

Sometimes inexperienced, young, or contract researchers have been pressured by their superiors to falsify or give a misleading interpretation of their results. It is far better to be honest than risk being associated with work that may subsequently be shown to be flawed. One strategy for avoiding such pressure is to keep good records.

20.4.2 Record keeping

Some research groups, especially in the biomedical sciences, are so concerned about honesty that they have a code of conduct where all researchers have to keep records of their ideas, hypotheses, methods, and results in hard bound laboratory books with numbered pages that are signed and dated on a daily or weekly basis by the researcher and their supervisor. Not only can these records be scrutinised if there is any doubt about the work (including who thought of something first), but it also encourages good data management and sequential record keeping. Results kept on pieces of loose paper with no reference to the methods used can be quite hard to interpret when the work is written up for publication.

20.5 Quality control in science

Publication in refereed journals ensures your work is scrutinised by at least one referee who is a specialist in the research field. Nevertheless, this process is more likely to detect obvious and inadvertent mistakes than deliberate dishonesty, and many journal editors have admitted that work they publish is likely to be flawed (LaFollette, 1992). Institutional strategies for quality control of the scientific process are becoming more common and many have rules about the storage and scrutiny of data. At the same time, however, there is a need in many institutions for explicit guidelines about the penalties for misconduct, together with mechanisms for handling alleged cases reported by others. The responsibility for doing good science is often left to the researcher and applies to every aspect of the scientific process, including devising logical hypotheses, doing well-designed experiments, and using and interpreting statistics appropriately, together with honesty, responsible and ethical behaviour, and fair dealing.

References

Andrews, M. L. A. (1976) *The Life that Lives On Man*. London: Faber & Faber.

Chalmers, A. F. (1999) *What Is This Thing Called Science?* 3rd edition. Indianapolis: Hackett Publishing Co.

Fisher, R. A. (1954) *Statistical Methods for Research Workers*. Edinburgh: Oliver & Boyd.

Hurlbert, S. J. (1984) Pseudoreplication and the design of ecological field experiments. *Ecological Monographs* **54**: 187–211.

Kuhn, T. S. (1970) *The Structure of Scientific Revolutions*, 2nd edition. Chicago: University of Chicago Press.

LaFollette, M. C. (1992) *Stealing into Print. Fraud, Plagiarism and Misconduct in Scientific Publishing*. Berkeley, CA: University of California Press.

Lakatos, I. (1978) The *Methodology of Scientific Research Programmes*. New York: Cambridge University Press.

McKillup, S. C. (1988) Behaviour of the millipedes. *Ommatoiulus moreletii*, *Ophyiulus verruciluger* and *Oncocladosoma castaneum* in response to visible light; an explanation for the invasion of houses by *Ommatoiulus moreletii*. *Journal of Zoology*, London **215**: 35–46.

McKillup, S. C. and McKillup, R. V. (1993) Behavior of the intertidal gastropod *Planaxis sulcatus* (Cerithiacae: Planaxidae) in Fiji: are responses to damaged conspecifics and predators more pronounced on tropical versus temperate shores? *Pacific Science* **47**: 401–7.

Popper, K. R. (1968) *The Logic of Scientific Discovery*. London: Hutchinson.

Quinn, G. P. and Keough, M. J. (2002) *Experimental Design and Data Analysis for Biologists*. Cambridge: Cambridge University Press.

Siegel, S. and Castallan, J. J. (1988) *Nonparametric Statistics for the Behavioral Sciences*. 2nd edition. New York: McGraw-Hill.

Singer, P. (1992) *Practical Ethics*. Cambridge: Cambridge University Press.

Sokal, R. R. and Rohlf, F. J. (1995) *Biometry*. 3rd edition. New York: W. H. Freeman.

Sprent, P. (1993) *Applied Nonparametric Statistical Methods*. 2nd edition. London: Chapman & Hall.

Student. (1908) The probable error of a mean. *Biometrica* **6**: 1–25.

Tukey, J. W. (1977) *Exploratory Data Analysis*. Reading: Addison Wesley.

Zar, J. H. (1999) *Biostatistical Analysis*, 3rd edition. Upper Saddle River, NJ: Prentice Hall.

Zelen, M. and Severo, N. C. (1964) Probability functions. In *Handbook of Mathematical Functions*, Abramowitz, M. and Stegun, I. (eds.). Washington, DC: National Bureau of Standards, pp. 925–95.

Index